AF735156

ATRIAL SEPTAL DEFECT

Edited by **P. Syamasundar Rao**

Atrial Septal Defect
Edited by P. Syamasundar Rao

Published by InTech
Janeza Trdine 9, 51000 Rijeka, Croatia

Copyright © 2012 InTech
All chapters are distributed under the Creative Commons Attribution 3.0 license, which allows users to download, copy and build upon published articles even for commercial purposes, as long as the author and publisher are properly credited, which ensures maximum dissemination and a wider impact of our publications. After this work has been published by InTech, authors have the right to republish it, in whole or part, in any publication of which they are the author, and to make other personal use of the work. Any republication, referencing or personal use of the work must explicitly identify the original source.

As for readers, this license allows users to download, copy and build upon published chapters even for commercial purposes, as long as the author and publisher are properly credited, which ensures maximum dissemination and a wider impact of our publications.

Notice
Statements and opinions expressed in the chapters are these of the individual contributors and not necessarily those of the editors or publisher. No responsibility is accepted for the accuracy of information contained in the published chapters. The publisher assumes no responsibility for any damage or injury to persons or property arising out of the use of any materials, instructions, methods or ideas contained in the book.

Publishing Process Manager Ivona Lovric

Technical Editor Teodora Smiljanic

Cover Designer InTech Design Team

Additional hard copies can be obtained from orders@intechopen.com

Atrial Septal Defect, Edited by P. Syamasundar Rao
p. cm.
ISBN 978-953-51-0531-2

We are IntechOpen, the world's leading publisher of Open Access books

Built by scientists, for scientists

4,100+
Open access books available

116,000+
International authors and editors

120M+
Downloads

151
Countries delivered to

Our authors are among the
Top 1%
most cited scientists

12.2%
Contributors from top 500 universities

BOOK CITATION INDEX
CLARIVATE ANALYTICS
INDEXED

WEB OF SCIENCE™

Selection of our books indexed in the Book Citation Index in Web of Science™ Core Collection (BKCI)

Interested in publishing with us?
Contact book.department@intechopen.com

Numbers displayed above are based on latest data collected.
For more information visit www.intechopen.com

For EU product safety concerns:
IN TECH d.o.o., Prolaz Marije Krucifikse Kozulić 3, 51000 Rijeka, Croatia,
info@intechopen.com or visit our website at intechopen.com.

Meet the editor

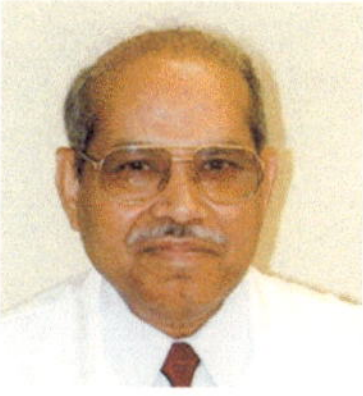

Dr P. Syamasundar Rao is Professor of Pediatrics and Medicine and Emeritus Chief of Pediatric Cardiology at the University of Texas-Houston Medical School and Professor of Pediatrics at the University Texas M.D. Anderson Cancer Center, Houston, Texas, USA. Dr. Rao received his medical degree from Andhra Medical College/University, Visakhapatnam. Following completion of pediatric training in USA, he received training in Pediatric Cardiology at Stanford University, Case-Western Reserve University and University of California at Los Angeles. After training he joined the faculty at the Medical College of Georgia, Augusta, Georgia, USA, then rose to the rank of Professor of Pediatrics and Associate Director of Pediatric Cardiology. Dr. Rao authored 350 papers, eight monographs/books and 55 book chapters.

Contents

Preface

Defects in the atrial septum are one the most common types of congenital heart defects (CHDs) in children and such a defect is the most common CHD in adults. Atrial septal defects (ASDs) cause left to right shunt because the left atrial pressure is higher than that in the right atrium. This causes volume overloading of the right ventricle. While this is generally well tolerated during infancy and childhood, development of exercise intolerance and arrhythmias in later childhood, adolescence and adulthood, and the risk for development of pulmonary vascular obstructive disease in adulthood make these defects important. The major types of atrial defects are ostium secundum, ostium primum, sinus venosus and coronary sinus ASDs and patent foramen ovale (PFO).

In the first chapter, I review the clinical features and management of ASDs. Patients with small defects are usually asymptomatic while moderate to large defects may present with symptoms. Physical findings include hyperdynamic precordium, widely split and fixed second heart sound, ejection systolic murmur at the left upper sternal border and a mid-diastolic flow rumble at the left lower sternal border. In patients with ostium primum ASDs, an apical holosystolic murmur may also be heard. Clinical diagnosis is not difficult and the diagnosis can be confirmed and quantified by echocardiographic studies. While surgical intervention was used in the past, transcatheter methods are currently used for closure of ostium secundum ASDs. Surgical correction is necessary for the ostium primum, sinus venosus and coronary sinus defects. PFO is present in nearly one third of normal population and is likely to be a normal variant and such isolated PFOs do not need intervention. When associated with other CHDs, the PFO facilitates intra-cardiac shunt to allow appropriate egress and/or mixing of blood flow. Hypoxemia in post-surgical residual defects including Fontan fenestrations, right ventricular infarction and platypnea-orthodexia syndrome may be secondary to right to left shunt across PFO and these defects may need closure. PFO, presumed to be the seat of paradoxical embolism resulting in stroke/transient ischemic attacks is the subject active investigation. Similarly the role of PFO in Caisson's disease and migraine is not well-established. There is varying degrees of evidence for benefit of transcatheter occlusion of these PFOs.

In the second chapter, Dr. Balaguru from the University of Texas Medical School, Houston, Texas discusses issues related to ASD in pregnant women. There are remarkable changes in cardiovascular physiology during pregnancy; the cardiac output increases, related to increased stroke volume and heart rate. The systemic vascular resistance decreases; however, concurrent increase in cardiac output keeps blood pressure stable. The blood volume increases (by 1.5 times) by raise in plasma volume; however, this is out of proportion to the increase in red cell mass with consequent relative anemia. These changes are tolerated well because the changes occur gradually. During the third trimester, enlarging uterus compresses the inferior vena cava (IVC) in supine posture leading to decrease in cardiac output and predisposes to deep vein thrombosis. In pregnant women with ASD, there is a greater increase in right atrial and right ventricular size (compared to pregnant women with no heart defect) and a higher incidence of supraventricular tachycardia. The probability of paradoxical embolism via the ASD is high given the predisposition to deep vein thrombosis and hypercoagulable state. If the diagnosis is known prior to pregnancy and the ASD is large and associated with moderate or severe right heart enlargement and is a potential candidate for supraventricular tachycardia and thromboembolic events during pregnancy, labor or postpartum, the ASD should be closed prior to planned-pregnancy. Transcatheter or surgical closure could be performed based on the size of the ASD and adequacy of septal rims. When the ASD is diagnosed during pregnancy but, the patient is asymptomatic without functional compromise (NYHA Class I and II) and has no heart failure, atrial arrhythmia, pulmonary hypertension or history of stroke, the these women are likely to do well throughout pregnancy and do not require transcatheter or surgical closure. On the contrary, in the presence of any of these issues, transcatheter or surgical closure may be performed. If transcatheter is opted, second trimester (13-28 weeks) is preferred instead of first trimester to avoid irradiation to the fetus. Local anesthesia with conscious sedation, intracardiac echocardiography to aid balloon sizing and device deployment and use of long venous sheath; the latter two to avoid or reduces radiation, may be appropriate. If the ASD is unsuitable for transcatheter closure, surgical closure of ASD may be performed in the second trimester with the following precautions: infusion of high-concentration of glucose (to provide energy for fetus), fetal monitoring, maintenance of high-flow, high mean arterial pressure (60 mmHg) and high hematocrit (> 25%) and hyper oxygenation. The author concludes that the need for closure of ASD during pregnancy is rare and if possible avoided. When closure is indicated transcatheter or surgical closure may be performed, taking appropriate precautions.

In the third chapter Reller from Oregon Health & Science University, Portland, Oregon reviews data on the prevalence, associated cardiac and non-cardiac findings and natural history of secundum ASDs, defined as size greater than 4 mm. The prevalence of secundum ASD is estimated to be 10.3 per 10,000 births, prevalence comparable to that of peri-membranous ventricular septal defects. The increase in the prevalence of secundum ASD was attributed to evaluation by color flow Doppler-echocardiography. The association of secundumASD with peri-membranous VSD and valvar pulmonary stenosis is well recognized. The cause(s) of secundum ASD remain largely unknown. Genetic syndromes associated with secundum ASD include Trisomy 21, 13 and 18;

Holt-Oram syndrome; chromosome 22q11 deletion in association with DiGeorge syndrome; velo-cardio-facial syndrome; Noonan syndrome and NKX2-5 gene defect. Patients with secundum ASD are more likely to have a positive family history of congenital heart disease. There is higher prevalence of secundum ASD in girls. Secundum ASD is also associated with non-cardiac malformations such as cleft palate and VACTERL association. Fetal alcohol syndrome, cytomegalovirus (CMV) and rubella infections during pregnancy and maternal diabetes are also associated with an increased prevalence of secundum ASD. Lower gestational age (low birth weight), small for gestational age, increased maternal age and multiple gestation pregnancy are also associated with higher prevalence of secundum ASD. With regard to natural history, the ASDs have a tendency to regress in size, including spontaneous closure. Small defects (between 4-5 mm) at the time of initial diagnosis either spontaneously close or regress to a size considered to be insignificant (≤ 3 mm). Larger defects (> 10 mm) do not close spontaneously and 75% of these patients may require surgical or device closure. It may be concluded that secundum ASD is the third most common congenital cardiac defect with incidence similar to peri-membranous VSD, the prevalence of secundum ASD is increasing, the cause of which remain speculative and there is a tendency for spontaneous closure or decreased size, especially in small defects.

Yamashita and associates from National Centre for Child Health and Development, Japan, in the chapter 4, describe a new approach with an automatic delivery system of high intensity focused ultrasound (HIFU) with real-time two dimensional-ultrasound (2D-US) imaging analysis to establish fetal interatrial communications. In the fetus with hypoplastic left heart syndrome (HLHS) and restrictive atrial septum leads to irreversible pulmonary vascular damage. The current approach of ultrasound-guided percutaneous puncture through both the uterine wall and fetal chest wall to create interatrial communications is associated with serious complications such as profound bradycardia, bleeding and hemopericardium and intracardiac thrombus formation. In addition, closure of the in utero created atrial septal defects can also occur prior to delivery. They developed a new approach with HIFU to establish fetal interatrial communications with potential for minimal adverse effects. HIFU ablation requires highly accurate pinpoint delivery in real-time based on computer-aided auto-tracking of atrial septum. Their system features automatic detection of rate of heart beat, automatic estimation of atrial septal position and automatic generation of HIFU delivery timing. They describe system configuration of computer-aided automatic HIFU delivery, automatic detection of heartbeat rates, position of the atrial septum and other procedural details. They performed a feasibility study for creation of an atrial septal defect using the beating heart of four anesthetized adult rabbits, which appear not to satisfactory. But, the authors interpret that they were able to confirm pinpoint delivery of HIFU to the pulsating atrial septum within beating hearts of anesthetized adult rabbits. The above studies were performed with 2D-US. Three-dimensional-US to track movement of intrauterine fetus may make the procedure more accurate. In conclusion, these workers developed computer-aided automatic delivery system of HIFU for creation of an atrial septal defect and further work to improve precision of the focus positioning of HIFU delivery and improvement of HIFU energy efficiency to intracardiac tissue is in progress. The concept appears good as is the design of the system. While the current results are far from clinically applicable, the technique has good potential.

In the fifth chapter from our institution, Alapati and I review the historical aspects of transcatheter closure of ASDs. Since the initial description of ASD occluding devices by King, Rashkind and their associates, a large number of single disc and double disc devices have been designed and tested in animal models followed by clinical trials in human subjects. Feasibility, safety and effectiveness have been demonstrated with most devices. However, design, redesign, testing and re-testing have been the typical path with most devices. Currently, only two devices are approved by the FDA in the US and these are: Amplatzer septal occluder and HELEX septal occluder. Several other devices are in development, some at the stage of animal experimentation and some in clinical trials in Europe or US. We will await for additional devices to be approved for general clinical use so that the practicing interventional cardiologist will have several devices at his/her disposal so that an appropriate device that suits best for a given patient and his/her defect is available. A brief review of historical aspects of PFO closure was also included. Majority of the ASD devices described in the ASD section, as and when they became available, have also been used to close PFOs; these include King's, clamshell, buttoned, Das-Angel-Wing and CardioSEAL devices. Existing devices were modified to address the anatomic features of the foramen ovale or new devices were designed to specifically address the PFOs and the latter include, Amplatzer PFO occluder, Cardia devices (PFO-Star and several of its subsequent generations), Premere occluder, Coherex Flat stent, PFx Closure System (not a device but employs monopolar radio frequency energy to effect closure of a PFO by welding the tissues of the septum primum with the septum secundum), pfm PFO-R, Solysafe PFO occluder and others. Amplatzer cribriform device was also used on off-label basis to close PFOs.

In the next chapter, Biliciler-Denktas, also from our institution, describes the role of transesophageal echocardiography (TEE) in percutaneous closure of ASDs. Initially the embryologic development of the atrial septum was reviewed. Currently used imaging techniques during device implantation, namely, transthoracic echocardiography, TEE, intracardiac echocardiography (ICE) and real time three-dimensional transesophageal echocardiography (3D TEE) were reviewed and relative advantages and disadvantages of each of these techniques were discussed; TEE and ICE are the two most commonly employed techniques. The importance of defined protocols to evaluate the heart, the atrial septal defect and the septal rims is stressed. Evaluation prior to device implantation include, examination of the entire atrial septum and its surrounding structures and exclusion of additional defects that may render the defect unsuitable for closure; measurement of the number and size of the defect(s); color Doppler imaging to define the shunt, left to right or right to left;

dimensions of the septal rims and measurement of balloon stretched diameter of the defect (when a sizing balloon is used) and identification of other defects while balloon occluding the defect. The echo and the interventional physicians work as a team to decide on the device size to be used for closure of ASD/PFO. Monitoring of the device deployment and verifying for correct position of the device prior to device release are germane. Post-implantation study will follow to detect impingement on valves, obstruction to venous return and residual shunting. TEE is also useful in the detection of complications of device closure such as device dislodgement and pericardial effusion/tamponade. The author concludes that TEE is of utmost value during percutaneous closure of ASDs and PFOs and is the preferred imaging modality in most catheterization laboratories.

In Chapter 7, Gonzalez and Hijazi of Rush University Medical Center, Chicago, Illinois, review the role of ICE in transcatheter closure of ASDs. Accurate and precise knowledge of the anatomy of the secundum ASD and the nearby structures is essential for safely performing ASD closure. While the conventional imaging method has been TEE, the authors advocate ICE to guide device closure of ASDs and PFOs because general anesthesia is not needed, risks of anesthesia are avoided and patient discomfort after the procedure is reduced. Ultrasound tipped catheters became available during the 1950s and 1960s and progressed thru' the current state of the art ICE catheters. several types of ICE catheters from different manufacturers are currently available and include, *UltraICE* mechanical single-element system (Boston Scientific Corp), *AcuNav* system (Siemens from Biosense-Webster), *ClearICE* system (St Jude Medical), *SoundStar* Catheter system (Biosense-Webster) and *ViewMate Z* Intracardiac Ultrasound System and *ViewFlex Plus* ICE Catheter (St Jude Medical). The authors opine that *AcuNav* catheter is the most popular ICE catheter currently in use. The AcuNav catheter should be carefully advanced from the groin to the heart under continuous fluoroscopic guidance to prevent inadvertent advancement of the catheter into side branches with potential vessel injury before reaching the right atrium. Their ICE protocol involves obtaining different views (home view, septal view, long axis view and short axis view) along with fluoroscopic images. Then ICE imaging during each step, namely, balloon sizing, deployment of left and then right disks and after releasing the device, is undertaken to ensure appropriate positioning of the device. The authors believe that ICE is more accurate in evaluation ASDs when compared to TEE, apart from avoiding general anesthesia, usually required for TEE. They mention limitations of ICE, which include large shaft size, complications related to ICE catheter placement, cost and non availability of real time three-dimensional (3D) imaging. They conclude that ICE along with fluoroscopy will improve the safety and outcome of percutaneous closure of ASDs.

In the next chapter, Sullebarger from Tampa, Florida, describes approaches to patients with technically challenging issues for transcatheter occlusion of ASDs and these include patients with poor femoral venous access, large defects and multiple defects. They also discuss minimally invasive, hybrid, transthoracic approach when percutaneous delivery of a device is not possible.

In the chapter 9, I address issues related why, when and how should ASDs be closed in adults. ASDs in adult subjects should be closed at presentation, electively, irrespective of their age. Evidence was presented to indicate that untreated ASD patients tend to have decreased event-free survival rates when compared to normal population and surgical closure is safe and effective with high event-free survival rates. ASD closure also prevents functional deterioration, improves cardiac function and increases functional capacity. Consequently hemodynamically significant (right ventricular volume overload) ASDs in adults should be occluded irrespective of symptomatology. When the effect of age at closure of ASD was examined, the Mayo Clinic data indicated that the actuarial survival rates are lower in patients who had surgery after 24 years of age; the earlier the surgery was performed the better were the 27-year survival rates. Since there is no advantage in waiting beyond 24 years of age, the closure should be performed at the time of identification of the case. While surgical closure is safe and effective, device closure has less morbidity, lower number of complications, requires less hospital stay and is less expensive than surgery. Multiple devices have been investigated over the last few decades, but only Amplatzer and HELEX devices received FDA approval as of this time. The Amplatzer is useful in most ASDs while the HELEX device is useful in small and medium-sized defects. Surgical repair is largely reserved for ASDs with poor septal rims. ASDs could also be closed surgically when intra-cardiac repair of other defects is contemplated. Some procedural details were mentioned with particular emphasis on the need for test occlusion of ASD in the elderly and testing with vasodilator agents in patients with associated pulmonary hypertension. Approaches taken to occlude ASDs with complex anatomy were also reviewed. Amplatzer device appears to be best available option for closure of ASDs at the present time. Careful attention to the details of the technique is mandatory to achieve successful outcomes.

In the next chapter Akagi of Okayama University Hospital, Okayama, Japan reviews ASD closure in geriatric population. He introduces the subject of ASDs in the elderly (≥ 70 years) by pointing out increasing prevalence of congenital heart disease in general and ASDs in particular in this age group. He also states that mortality of congenital heart disease in the aged is increasing during past few decades. The clinical features of ASD in the elderly are different from those in children and young adults because they present with hemodynamic abnormalities such as pulmonary hypertension, valvar regurgitation, congestive heart failure and left ventricular diastolic dysfunction, atrial arrhythmias and co-morbidities, such as hypertension, chronic obstructive lung disease, coronary artery disease, kidney disease and others. The author emphasizes that there are only a few studies in the aged population re functional results of catheter and surgical closure of ASD and reviews his experience with catheter closure of ASD in geriatric patients as well as long-term outcome. Of the 420 patients who had attempted transcatheter closure of ASD at their institution, 30 patients were older than 70 years. Their mean age was 75.8 ± 3.8 years with a range of 70 and 85 years. Mean ASD diameter was 20.3 ± 6.4 mm and mean pulmonary-systemic flow (Qp/Qs) was 2.4 ± 0.7. Test balloon occlusion of ASD with measurement of pulmonary arterial wedge pressure was performed in only 7 of 30 cases. Device implantation was successful in 28 (93%) of the 30 patients. Significant improvement of NYHA functional class in 20 (74%) of the 27 patients, significant improvement in plasma BNP level, decreased resting heart rate, improvement of tricuspid regurgitation in 11 of 17 patients (65%) and cardiac remodeling with improvement in RVEDD/LVEDD ratio at follow-up were observed. The author concludes that their experience in the elderly patients, while small, indicates that transcatheter closure of ASD can be performed safely and contributes to improvement of NYHA functional class and encourages positive cardiac remodeling.

In the Chapter 11, Numan from the University of Texas Medical School, Houston discusses the role of ASD/PFO in migraine. The incidence of migraine is 13% and has adverse affect on social life and potential for development of neurological complications. The age of migraine attacks is said to 20 to 64 years with the majority occurring prior to the age of 30 years. Migraine with aura, also known as "classic migraine" is seen in only 25% cases. There is an increased prevalence of PFOs in patients with migraine, but no causal relationship between these two is established. Such association appears to more convincing in patients with migraine with aura. The author then describes the pathologic anatomy and echocardiographic features of PFO. Transcranial Doppler has higher sensitivity than Echo (TTE, TEE or ICE) in detecting the right to left shunt across the PFO. The author reviews several studies examining the effect of occlusion of PFOs with devices; most single institutional, non-randomized studies show improvement in migraine; this improvement is greater in patients with aura. However, Migraine Intervention With STARFlex Technology (MIST), a randomized prospective study with patients blinded for PFO closure did not demonstrate statistical difference between the two groups. The author offers several objections to the interpretation of the study, but concludes that the MIST study raises questions to be addressed in future studies. However, it may be concluded that the majority of the studies show benefit to patients suffering from migraine with aura.

In the last chapter, Daraban and her associates, also from the University of Texas Medical School, Houston discusses transcatheter occlusion of atrial defects for prevention of recurrence of paradoxical embolism. Stroke is the third most common cause of death in the United States. Cryptogenic stroke, consisting of 40% of stroke population may be related paradoxical embolism via PFO or ASD. Therapeutic measures for secondary prevention in this patient population include medical treatment or surgical/percutaneous closure of the PFO/ASD. The authors describe embryology, fetal and postnatal changes of PFO. The authors then describe the anatomy and associated anomalies such as atrial septal aneurysms (ASA), Chiari network and fenestrated atrial septum. TEE with or without contrast injection and Valsalva maneuver and transcranial Doppler (TCD) are important diagnostic tools in the identification of right-to-left shunt across the PFO. They then go on to describe the rationale for PFO and ASD closure treatment in patients with paradoxical embolism. The authors briefly describe the devices used for occlusion of PFO and describe in detail the procedure of closure using Amplatzer PFO Occluder. A number of randomized clinical studies comparing medical treatment with closure of atrial defect are underway. The authors describe the CLOSURE I, REDUCE and RESPECT trials. CLOSURE I, a randomized trial compared the safety and efficacy of percutaneous PFO closure with STARFlex device versus best medical therapy. During a two year follow-up, the rates of stroke or transient ischemic attack (TIA) were no different between groups. REDUCE is a FDA approved prospective, randomized, multicenter trial designed to demonstrate the safety and effectiveness of the HELEX Septal Occluder for PFO closure in patients with a history of cryptogenic stroke or TIA. The RESPECT trial is a randomized, multi-center study investigating whether closure of PFOs using the Amplatzer PFO Occluder device is safer and more effective than current standard-of-care treatment in the prevention of a cryptogenic stroke. If the results of these clinical trials, favor device closure, it is likely that percutaneous PFO closure can be used to prevent recurrence of paradoxical embolism and stroke.

Of the major types of atrial defects, namely ostium secundum, ostium primum, sinus venosus and coronary sinus ASDs and PFO, ostium primum, sinus venosus and coronary sinus defects usually require surgical closure. Such surgery may be performed at about 3 to 4 years of age or if they present later, at the time of presentation. Earlier surgery is not necessary unless heart failure is present. Ostium secundum ASDs can be successfully closed with transcatheter methodology and the majority of the book addresses the issues related such technology. PFOs are ordinarily considered as normal variants, although, sometimes they become the seat of right left shunting, requiring closure. The evidence for closure PFO with potential right to left shunt in situations related to paradoxical embolism, migraine and others is equivocal. The studies currently in progress may throw light on this subject. While the majority of the book addresses closure of atrial septal defects, one chapter in particular focuses on creating atrial defects in the fetus with HLHS. I hope that the fund of information provided in this book will be use to the practicing physician caring for infants, children and adults with suspected or known ASDs which may aid them in providing optimal care for their patients.

Dr. P. Syamasundar Rao
University of Texas at Houston Medical School
Houston, Texas,
USA

Section 1

General Review of Atrial Septal Defects

1

Atrial Septal Defect – A Review

P. Syamasundar Rao
University of Texas at Houston Medical School, Houston, Texas, USA

1. Introduction

Defects in the atrial septum cause left to right shunt because the left atrial pressure is higher than that in the right atrium. This causes volume overloading of the right ventricle. While this is generally well tolerated in infancy and childhood, development of exercise intolerance and arrhythmias in later childhood and adolescence, and the risk for development of pulmonary vascular obstructive disease in adulthood make these defects important. There are four major types of atrial septal defects (ASDs) and these include ostium secundum, ostium primum, sinus venosus and coronary sinus defects. The clinical features are essentially similar and I will present detailed discussion of ostium secundum and primum ASDs followed by brief presentation of the other two defects.

Persistent patency of the foramen ovale in nearly one third of normal population makes the patent foramen ovale (PFO) a normal variant, although these become important in the presence of other structural abnormalities of the heart and when they become the seat of right to left shunt causing paradoxical embolism resulting in stroke/transient ischemic attacks or other problems, such as migraine, Caisson's disease and platypnea-orthodexia syndrome. The issues related these types of PFOs will be briefed at the conclusion of this chapter.

2. Secundum atrial septal defect

Atrial septal defects constitute 8% to 13% of all congenital heart defects (CHDs). Pathologically, there is deficiency of the septal tissue in the region of fossa ovalis. These may be small to large. Most of the time, these are single defects, although, occasionally multiple defects and fenestrated defects can also be seen. Because of left-to-right shunting across the defects, the right atrium and right ventricle are dilated and somewhat hypertrophied. Similarly, main and branch pulmonary arteries are also dilated. Pulmonary vascular obstructive changes are not usually seen until adulthood.

Mitral valve abnormalities, including mitral valve prolapse and mitral insufficiency may be seen in some patients. It is not clear whether these abnormalities are to due to right ventricular volume overloading or intrinsic abnormality of the mitral valve. Pulmonary valvar pressure gradients are seen frequently and are thought to be related to increased flow and/or differences in expression of kinetic and potential energies in the right ventricle and pulmonary artery (Rao et al 1973); however, true pulmonary stenosis is present in only 5% of ASD patients. Persistent left superior vena cava may be present in 10% patients.

2.1 Clinical features

The clinical features are essentially similar in all types of ASDs mentioned in the Introduction section.

2.1.1 Symptoms

Isolated ASD patients are usually asymptomatic and are most often detected at the time of preschool physical examination. Sometimes these defects are detected when echocardiographic studies are performed for some unrelated reason. A few patients do present with symptoms of heart failure in infancy, although this is uncommon.

2.1.2 Physical examination

The right ventricular and right ventricular outflow tract impulses are increased and hyperdynamic. No thrills are usually felt. The second heart sound is widely split and fixed (splitting does not vary with respiration) and is the most characteristic sign of ASD. Ejection systolic clicks are rare with ASDs. The ejection systolic murmur of ASD is soft and is of grade I-II/VI intensity and rarely, if ever, louder. The murmur is secondary to increased blood flow across the pulmonary valve and is heard best at the left upper sternal border. A grade I-II/VI mid-diastolic flow rumble is heard (with the bell of the stethoscope) best at the left lower sternal border. This is due to large volume flow across the tricuspid valve. There is no audible murmur because of flow across the ASD.

2.2 Noninvasive evaluation

2.2.1 Chest x-ray

Chest film usually reveals mild to moderate cardiomegaly, prominent main pulmonary artery segment and increased pulmonary vascular markings.

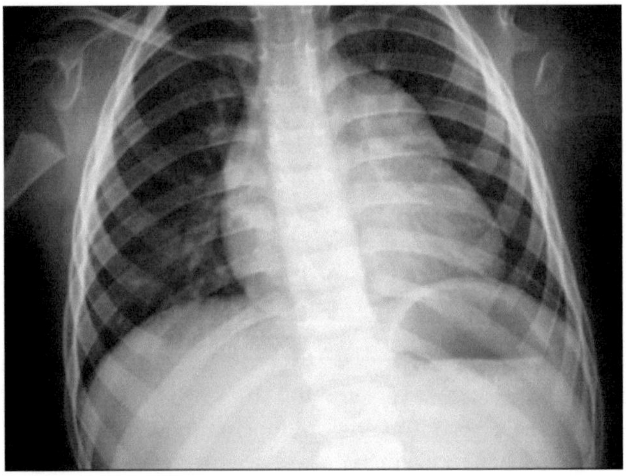

Fig. 1. Chest x-ray in posterior-anterior view demonstrating mild cardiomegaly, increased pulmonary vascular markings and a slightly prominent main pulmonary artery segment as seen in patients with atrial septal defect.

2.2.2 Electrocardiogram

The ECG shows mild right ventricular hypertrophy; the so-called diastolic volume overload pattern with rsR' pattern in the right chest leads.

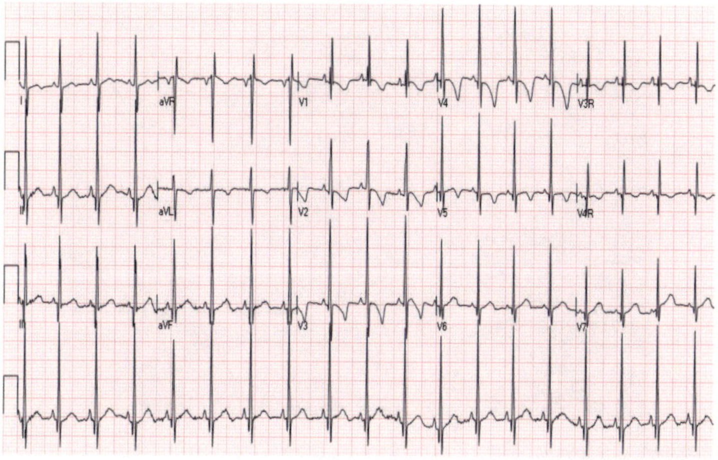

Fig. 2. An electrocardiogram demonstrating rsR′ pattern in right chest leads, the so called diastolic overloading pattern, indicative mild right ventricular hypertrophy, seen in patients with atrial septal defects.

2.2.3 Echocardiogram

Echocardiographic studies reveal enlarged right ventricle with paradoxical septal motion, particularly well-demonstrable on M-mode echocardiograms in patients with moderate to large ASDs. Dilatation of the right ventricle may not be present in small defects. By two-dimensional echocardiogram, the defect can be clearly visualized (Figure 3 left panel).

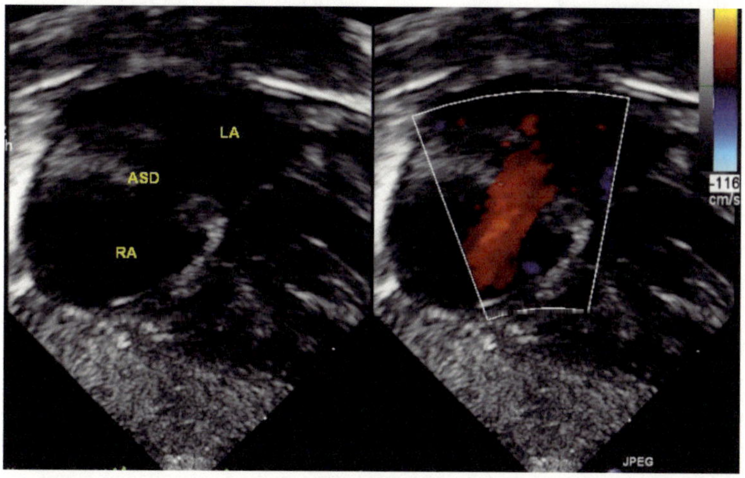

Fig. 3. Two dimensional subcostal echocardiographic views of the atrial septum demonstrating secundum atrial septal defect (ASD) in the mid septum (left panel) and color Doppler with left to right shunt (right panel). LA, left atrium; RA, right atrium.

The type of ASD, ostium secundum (Figure 3) versus ostium primum (Figure 4) can also be delineated by the echocardiographic study.

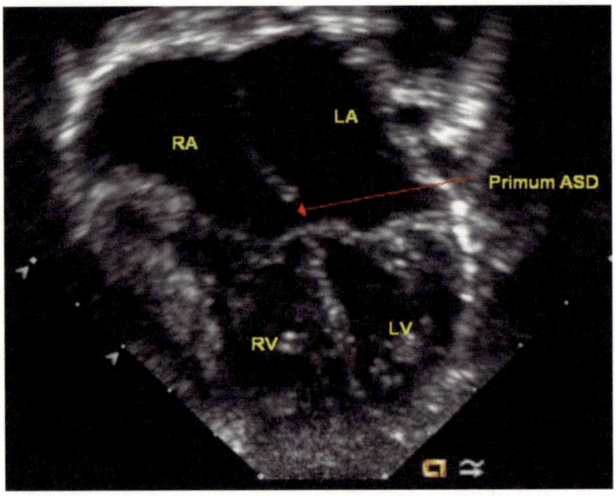

Fig. 4. Four chambered view of the heart demonstrates ostium primum atrial septal defect (ASD), arrow. Note absence of any atrial septal tissue superior to the crest of the ventricular septum. The right atrium (RA) and right ventricle (RV) are enlarged. LA, left atrium; LV. left ventricle.

Apical and precordial views may show "septal drop-outs" without an ASD because of thinness of the septum in the region of fossa ovalis. Therefore, subcostal views should be scrutinized for evidence of ASD. In addition, demonstration of flow across the defect with pulsed Doppler and color Doppler (Figure 3, right panel) echocardiography is necessary to avoid false positive studies. In adolescents and adults transesophageal echo (TEE) is needed to make definitive diagnosis of ASD. (Figures 5 and 6)

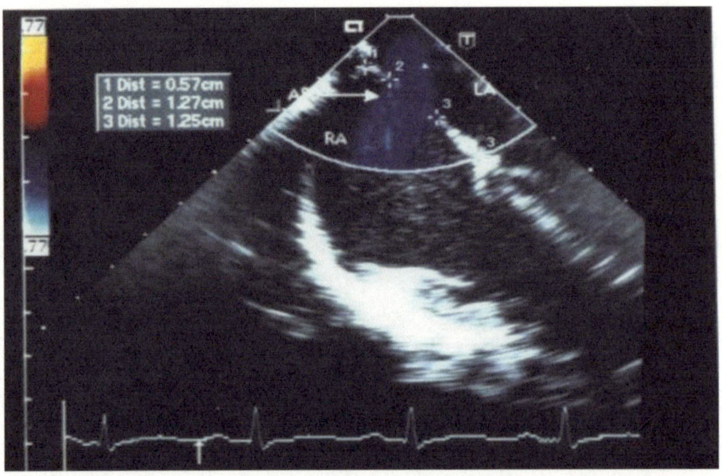

Fig. 5. Selected two-dimensional and color flow frame from a transesophageal echocardiographic (TEE) study (in adult patient) of the atrial septum shows an atrial septal defect (arrow) with left to right shunt (blue flow). Measurements of septal margins (1 Dist and 3 Dist) and of the defect (2 Dist) are shown in the insert. LA, left atrium; RA, right atrium.

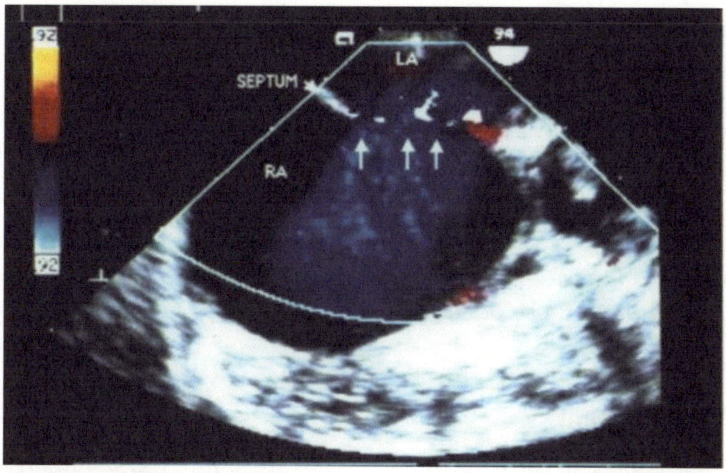

Fig. 6. Selected two-dimensional and color flow frame from a transesophageal echocardiographic (TEE) study (in another adult patient) of the atrial septum shows multi-fenestrated atrial septal defect (arrows) with left to right shunt (blue flow). LA, left atrium; RA, right atrium.

2.2.4 Other imaging studies

Other imaging studies such as three-dimensional echo, MRI and CT can and do demonstrate the defect, but are not necessary for routine cases.

2.3 Catheterization and angiography

Clinical and echocardiographic features are sufficiently characteristic so that cardiac catheterization is not necessary for the diagnosis. However, cardiac catheterization is an integral part of transcatheter occlusion of the ASD.

When catheterization is performed, one will observe step-up in oxygen saturation at the right atrial level. The right ventricular or pulmonary arterial saturations may be better to estimate the degree of shunting because of improved mixing in these distal sites. The pulmonary venous, left atrial, left ventricular and aortic saturations are within normal range. In large defects, the pressures in both atria are equal while in small defects, an inter-atrial pressure difference is noted. The right ventricular and pulmonary arterial pressures are usually normal during childhood. Calculated pulmonary-to-systemic flow ratio (Qp:Qs) is used to quantify the degree of shunting and a Qp:Qs in excess of 1.5:1 is considered an indication for closure of ASD.

Selective cineangiography in the right upper pulmonary vein at its junction with the left atrium in a left axial oblique view will reveal location and the size of the ASD. When anomalous pulmonary venous connection is suspected, selective left or right pulmonary arterial angiography should be performed and the levophase of angiogram should be scrutinized for anomalous pulmonary venous connections.

To avoid missing a diagnosis of partial anomalous pulmonary venous return, we usually perform a number of routine maneuvers and these include (i) measurement of oxygen saturations from both right and left innominate veins at the time of superior vena caval sampling, (ii) left innominate vein cineangiogram in posterior-anterior view with diluted contrast material, (iii) probe for all the four pulmonary veins from the left atrium and (iv) as mentioned before, obtain cineangiography from the right upper pulmonary vein at its junction with the left atrium in a left axial oblique (30^0 LAO and 30^0 cranial) view.

2.4 Management

The management of ASD patients is largely dependent of the age at presentation, presence of symptoms, particularly those of congestive heart failure and the size of the defect (and magnitude of the shunt).

2.4.1 Medical management

As mentioned earlier, congestive heart failure is rare with ASDs, although occasionally, failure symptoms may be present in infancy. In these infants anti-congestive measures (diuretics and digoxin) should be instituted. If they do not improve, surgical and more recently trans-catheter intervention to close the defects are considered.

Small ASDs, not requiring closure may be followed at infrequent intervals. SBE prophylaxis and activity restriction are not generally recommended for ASD patients.

2.4.2 Indications for closure

Despite lack of symptoms at presentation, closure of moderate to large ASDs is recommended so as to 1) prevent development of pulmonary vascular obstructive disease later in life, 2) reduce chances for supra-ventricular arrhythmias and 3) prevent development of symptoms during adolescence and adulthood. Elective closure around age 4 to 5 years is recommended. Closure during infancy is not undertaken unless the infant is symptomatic. Right ventricular volume overloading by echocardiogram and a Qp:Qs >1.5 (if the child had cardiac catheterization) are indications for closure.

2.4.3 Surgical management

Following the introduction of cardiopulmonary bypass techniques for open heart surgery and the description of surgical closure of ASD by Gibbon, Lillehei and Kirklin in 1950s, it rapidly became a standard treatment for atrial defects. The conventional treatment of choice of moderate and large defects until recently is surgical correction. Under general anesthesia, a median sternotomy or a right submammary incision is made, the aorta and vena cavae are cannulated and the patient placed on cardiopulmonary bypass. Right atriatomy is made and the defect exposed and closed either by approximating the defect margins with suture material or by using a pericardial patch, depending upon the size of the defect.

While surgical closure of ostium secundum ASDs is safe and effective with low (<1%) mortality, the morbidity associated with sternotomy/thoracotomy, cardiopulmonary bypass and potential for postoperative complications cannot be avoided. Other disadvantages of surgical therapy are the expense associated with surgical correction, residual surgical scar and psychological trauma to the patients and/or the parents. Because of these reasons several trans-catheter methods have been developed (Chopra and Rao, 2000; Rao, 2003) which will be reviewed in the next section.

At the present time, surgical repair is largely reserved for defects with poor septal rims in which the interventional cardiologist deems that defect is difficult to close with trans-catheter methodology or was unsuccessful in closing the defect. Also, if intra-cardiac repair of other defects is contemplated, surgical closure of ASD could be performed at the same time.

2.4.4 Trans-catheter closure

As alluded to above, a large number of devices have been developed over the last three and one-half decades. Some of the devices have been discontinued and others modified and redesigned (Rao, 1998; Rao, 2000; Rao, 2003b). Clinical trials have been undertaken with a large number of devices as reviewed elsewhere (Rao, 2000; Rao, 2003b) and feasibility, safety and effectiveness of these devices in occluding the ASD have been demonstrated.

Clinical trials have been undertaken in a large number of patients with Bard clamshell septal occluder and buttoned device and feasibility and effectiveness of these devices in occluding the ASD have been demonstrated. Fractures of one or more arms of the clamshell device with occasional embolization, has prompted the investigators and the US Food and Drug Administration (FDA) to withdraw the device from clinical trials. The buttoned device has undergone clinical trials and, immediate and short-term follow-up results are encouraging (Rao et al 1992, Rao et al 1994, Rao et al 2000, Rao and Sideris 2001). However, pre-market-approval (PMA) application was not made and consequently it is not approved by the FDA and is not available for general clinical use. Subsequently, a large number of other devices (Das Angel-Wing, ASDOS, Amplatzer, CardioSeal, HELEX and others) have been introduced and clinical trials began (Chopra and Rao 2000). At the present time however, Amplatzer Septal Occluder and HELEX are the only two devices that are approved for general clinical use by the FDA. The experience with Amplatzer for most defects has been encouraging. HELEX device is only useful in small to medium-sized defects. A number of other devices are in clinical trials either in the US or in other countries with local, national or regional IRB supervision. These devices, to the best of my knowledge, are CardioSeal/StarFlex devices, transcatheter patch, pfm ASD-R device, bio-absorbable NMT devices (Bio-STAR and Bio-TREK), Occlutech Flex device, Cardia devices (INTRASEPT, ATRIASEPT I/II-ASD and ULTRASEPT), Solysafe Septal Occluder, Heart R Septal Occluder (manufactured in China) and others. The Amplatzer Septal Occluder is rapidly becoming the device of choice because of ease with which the device can be implanted, retrieved and repositioned plus the comfort that the device is FDA approved.

2.4.4.1 Amplatzer septal occluder

Amplatzer septal occluder is a double disk device constructed with 0.004" to 0.007" Nitinol (nickle-titanium compound) wire with shape memory. A 4 mm wide waist connects the left and right atrial disks and stents the ASD. The left atrial disk is slightly larger than the right. Dacron polyester patches are sewn into each disk. Multiple sizes are available from the manufacturer (AGA); the device size is expressed as the size of waist of the device. The device can be withdrawn into a delivery sheath and can be implanted across the defect and if necessary pulled back into the sheath and repositioned.

2.4.4.1.1 Method of device implantation

The procedure involves percutaneous right heart catheterization to confirm the clinical and echocardiographic diagnosis with particular attention to exclude partial anomalous pulmonary venous return. A left atrial cineangiogram in a left axial oblique view (30^0 LAO and 30^0 Cranial) with the catheter positioned in the right upper pulmonary vein at its junction with the left atrium is then performed. This is followed by transesophageal (TEE) or intracardiac (ICE) echocardiography to measure the size of the ASD, to visualize entry of all pulmonary veins into the left atrium and to examine the atrial septal rims. Static balloon sizing of the ASD using NuMed PTS or AGA Amplatzer sizing balloons is performed routinely by some cardiologists. During balloon occlusion, color Doppler evaluation of the atrial septum to rule out additional atrial defects should be carried out. However, I do not routinely perform balloon sizing, but rely on the TEE sizing; I utilize the thick margins of the defect to measure the size of the ASD, leaving out the flail margins, a method similar to that suggested by Carcagnì and Presbitero (2004).

An Amplatzer Septal Occluder that is 1 to 2 mm larger than the diameter of the ASD is selected for implantation. The size of delivery sheath accommodating the selected device is then be positioned in the left upper pulmonary vein, taking appropriate precautions to avoid inadvertent air entry into the system. The selected device is screwed onto the delivery cable; the device is loosened by unscrewing by one turn and drawn into the loader sheath under saline. The device is deposited into the delivery sheath while flushing the loader sheath continuously with saline or a similar flushing solution. This is to prevent inadvertent air entry into the system. The device is advanced within the sheath under fluoroscopic guidance until it reaches the tip of the delivery sheath in the left upper pulmonary vein. It is important not to rotate the delivery cable to prevent inadvertent unscrewing of the device. The entire system is withdrawn until the tip of the sheath slips into the free left atrium and the device advanced, thus releasing the left atrial disk. Under echocardiographic guidance, the entire system is withdrawn such that the left atrial disk is flush against the left atrial side of the atrial septum occluding the ASD. Then, while the device cable is held steady, the delivery sheath is withdrawn releasing the waist of the device within the atrial septal defect, followed by further withdrawal of the sheath deploying the right atrial disk in the right atrium. The position of the device is verified by echocardiography and residual shunt looked for. If the device position is satisfactory, the device cable is moved back and forth (so called Minnesota Wiggle). The position of the device is again verified by TEE (or ICE). If the device position is unsatisfactory, the device can be withdrawn into the sheath and redeployed. Then the device cable is rotated counterclockwise, releasing the device. A repeat TEE to ensure good position of the device is undertaken. Right atrial cineangiography through the delivery sheath is performed by some cardiologists prior to withdrawal of the delivery sheath out of body.

Arterial line to monitor the systemic pressures throughout the procedure, administration of heparin (100 units/kg) and monitoring the ACT to keep it above 200 seconds, and administration of Ancef or a similar antibiotic are routine parts of the procedure. Aspirin 5 mg/kg as a single daily dose for six months is usually recommended. Clopidogrel (Plavix) is used in adult patients.

2.4.4.1.2 Complex defects

Large defects, small septal rims, multiple defects and septal aneurysms pose additional problems and appropriate adjustments in the technique (Nagm and Rao 2004) should be undertaken to ensure success of the device implantation.

2.4.4.1.3 Results

Both immediate and mid-term follow-up results of Amplatzer Septal Occluder appear excellent with immediate complete closure rates varying from 62% to 96% which improved to 83% to 99% at six to 12 month follow-up (Hamdan et al 2003). We undertook closure of 80 ostium secundum defects with this device; there was a small residual shunt in two patients at the conclusion of the procedure. This shunt disappeared at one and six month follow-up visits respectively. No residual shunts were observed during a mean follow-up of 24 months.

2.4.4.2 HELEX device

HELEX device is constructed with a single stand super-elastic, Nitinol wire frame with ultrathin poly-tetra-fluro-ethelene (ePTFE) covering the entire length of the wire; the device can be loaded into a 9-F delivery sheath. The delivery system has three components, a delivery catheter, control catheter and a mandrel. When deployed, it forms two interconnected round disks, designed to be placed on either side of the atrial septum. The device is available in 15 thru' 35 mm diameter sizes in 5 mm increments.

2.4.4.2.1 Method of device implantation

The procedures of catheterization and defect sizing are similar those described in Amplatzer device section. The method of implantation is detailed elsewhere (Latson et al 2003). In brief, the delivery catheter (Green) is placed in the left atrium over a guide wire and the wire removed. Push-pinch-pull method is used to form the left atrial disk and the disk pulled back gently to engage the left side of the atrial septum, under fluoroscopic and/or TEE or ICE guidance. Then the delivery (Green) catheter is withdrawn over the control (Gray) catheter until the mandrel (Tan) engages the hub. Then the green catheter is held study while the gray catheter is advanced to deliver the right atrial disk on the right atrial side of the septum, again using the "push-pinch-pull" technique. Once the device position is verified by echocardiography (TEE or ICE), the device is locked and then released. Intra and post procedural management is similar to that described in the Amplatzer device section.

2.4.4.2.2 Results

Results of the multicenter trial (Jones et al 2007) suggest successful implantation in 87% patients with low incidence of residual leaks (2.6% at one year follow-up) and modest incidence (8%) of wire frame fractures. It is generally considered to be a good device for occlusion of small to medium-sized ASDs.

2.5 Prognosis

The prognosis following surgical or transcatheter closure of ASDs is excellent, provided that they do not have pulmonary hypertension or atrial tachycardia. Actuarial survival rate following surgery were 97%, 90%, 83% and 74% at 5, 10, 20 and 30 years respectively (Murphy et al 1990) and were slightly worse than that of control (normal) population (99%,

98%, 94% & 85%). However, if surgical correction is performed prior to 25 years of age, the actuarial survival rates are similar to normal population. Similar favorable results can be expected if the defect is closed by trans-catheter methodology prior to 25 years of age.

3. Ostium primum ASDs

Ostium primum ASDs belong to the group of defects called atrio-ventricular septal defects (AVSDs) and are thought to be caused by defective embryonic development of embryonic endocardial cushions. There is persistence of the embryonic ostium primum, located in the posterior portion of the lower part of the atrial septum, usually large in size. A cleft in the anterior leaflet of the mitral valve is present, causing mitral insufficiency of varying degree. Depending upon the direction of mitral insufficiency jet, there may be a left ventricular-to-right atrial shunt as well. A cleft in the septal leaflet of the tricuspid valve may be present in some patients. These defects are formerly known as partial endocardial cushion defects. These defects are also called partial AVSDs; this is in contradistinction to complete AVSDs in which atrial and ventricular septal defects and clefts in the mitral and tricuspid valves with common atrio-ventricular valve are present. There may be associated ostium secundum ASD, patent foramen ovale or a persistent left superior vena cava draining into the coronary sinus.

The left ventricular outflow tract is long and narrow and sometimes the abnormal attachments of the atrio-ventricular valve tissue may cause left ventricular outflow tract obstruction.

Dilatation of the right heart structures is similar to that described for ostium secundum atrial septal defects. In the presence moderate to severe mitral insufficiency left ventricular dilatation may also be present.

3.1 Clinical features

The clinical features are essentially similar to that described for ostium secundum ASDs; however in the presence of significant mitral insufficiency symptoms of heart failure may be present.

3.1.1 Symptoms

Isolated ostium primum ASD patients are usually asymptomatic and are most often detected at the time of preschool physical examination. However, murmurs associated with mitral insufficiency of ostium primum defects may also result in early detection of these defects. A few patients do present with symptoms of heart failure in infancy or childhood especially in the presence of significant mitral insufficiency.

3.1.2 Physical examination

The right ventricular and right ventricular outflow tract impulses are increased and hyperdynamic. No thrills are usually felt. The second heart sound is widely split and fixed (splitting does not vary with respiration) and is the most characteristic sign of ASD. Ejection systolic clicks are rare with ASDs. The ejection systolic murmur of ASD is soft and is of grade I-II/VI intensity and rarely, if ever, louder. The murmur is secondary to increased blood flow across the pulmonary valve and is heard best at the left upper sternal border. A grade I-II/VI mid-diastolic flow rumble is heard (with the bell of the stethoscope) best at the left lower sternal border. This is due to large volume flow across the tricuspid valve. There is no audible murmur because of flow across the ASD. A holosystolic murmur of mitral insufficiency is heard best at the apex with radiation into the anterior and/or mid axillary line. A grade I-II/VI mid-diastolic flow rumble, heard best at the apex may be appreciated in the presence significant mitral insufficiency. Signs of heart failure may be present in cases with severe mitral insufficiency.

3.2 Noninvasive evaluation

3.2.1 Chest x-ray

Chest film usually reveals mild to moderate cardiomegaly, prominent main pulmonary artery segment and increased pulmonary vascular markings. In the presence of significant mitral insufficiency, the cardiomegaly may be more prominent.

3.2.2 Electrocardiogram

Prolongation of PR interval (first degree heart block) is commonly seen. Right atrial, left atrial or biatrial enlargement is seen nearly half of the patients. The ECG also shows mild right ventricular hypertrophy; the so-called diastolic volume overload pattern with rsR' pattern in the right chest leads. Left ventricular hypertrophy may be seen if there is significant mitral insufficiency. Characteristically, the mean frontal plane vector is oriented superiorly between -30^{0} and -90^{0}, the so called left axis deviation and this is typical for endocardial cushion defects.

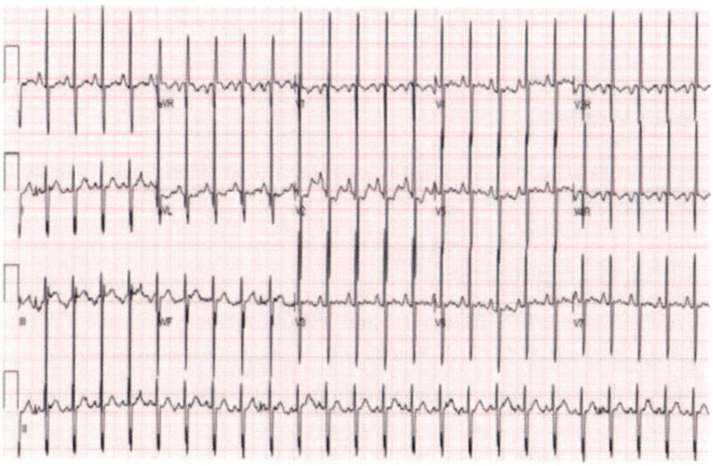

Fig. 7. An electrocardiogram of a child with ostium primum atrial septal defect demonstrating left axis deviation (-45^{0} - deep S waves in leads II, III and AVF), right atrial enlargement (tall P waves in leads I and V2) and right ventricular hypertrophy (tall R waves in lead V2 and deep S waves in leads V5 and V6).

3.2.3 Echocardiogram

Echocardiographic studies reveal enlarged right ventricle with paradoxical septal motion, particularly well-demonstrable on M-mode echocardiograms in patients with moderate to large ASDs. By two-dimensional echocardiogram, the defect can be clearly visualized (Figure 4). The type of ASD, secundum versus primum can also be delineated by the echocardiographic study (Figure 3 & 4). Demonstration of flow across the defect with color Doppler (Figure 8) echocardiography is possible. Cleft in the mitral valve may be demonstrated in precordial short axis views and mitral insufficiency jet may be shown in four chamber views (Figure 8).

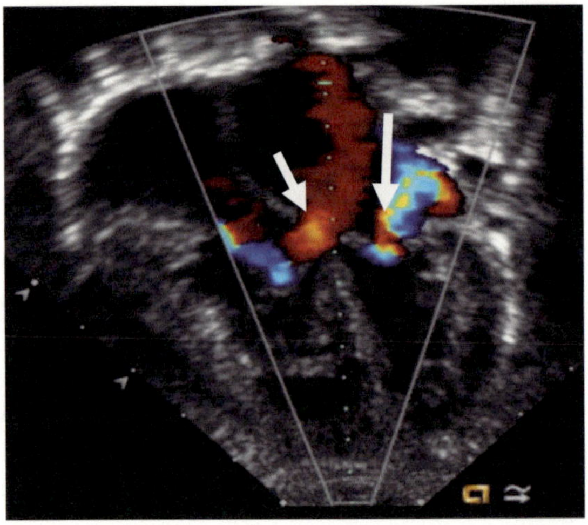

Fig. 8. Four chambered view of the heart demonstrates left-to-right shunt (red flow) across the ostium primum atrial septal defect (short arrow). Also note mitral insufficiency (long arrow).

3.2.4 Other imaging studies

Other imaging studies such as three-dimensional echo, MRI and CT may also demonstrate the defects, but are not necessary for routine cases.

3.3 Catheterization and angiography

Clinical and echocardiographic features are characteristic for the defect and cardiac catheterization is not necessary for the diagnosis. If pulmonary hypertension is suspected or if there are issues that can't be resolved by echocardiography, catheterization may be undertaken.

If catheterization is performed, step-up in oxygen saturation at the right atrial level is seen. The left heart saturations are within normal range. Because the defects are usually large, the mean pressures in both atria are equal. The right ventricular and pulmonary arterial pressures are usually normal during childhood. The left heart pressures are also normal unless there is left ventricular outflow tract obstruction. Calculated pulmonary-to-systemic flow ratio (Qp:Qs) is used to quantify the degree of shunting and the Qp:Qs is usually in excess of 2:1. Pulmonary vascular resistance is usually normal.

Selective left ventricular cineangiography reveals a long and narrow left ventricular outflow tract resulting in what is described as goose-neck deformity, characteristic of endocardial cushion defects.

3.4 Management

The management of ostium primum ASD patients is largely dependent of the age at presentation and presence of symptoms, particularly those of congestive heart failure.

3.4.1 Medical management

Congestive heart failure is rare with ostium primum ASDs, although failure symptoms may be present in the presence of significant mitral insufficiency. In these patients anti-congestive measures (diuretics and digoxin) should be instituted. If they do not improve, surgical closure should be considered.

Transcatheter occlusion, now a standard treatment for ostium secundum ASDs, is not feasible in patients with ostium primum ASDs because there are no inferior septal rims, but more importantly because the need for addressing mitral valve cleft and the accompanying mitral insufficiency.

SBE prophylaxis is recommended and normal activity is permitted in the absence of severe mitral insufficiency.

3.4.2 Indications for closure

Although surgical correction can be performed at any age, surgery in asymptomatic patients is usually recommended at the age of 3 to 4 years. In the presence of symptoms or if there is associated severe mitral insufficiency, surgical repair may be performed at presentation, after medically controlling the heart failure.

3.4.3 Surgical management

The conventional treatment of choice of ostium primum ASDs is surgical correction. Under general anesthesia, a median sternotomy incision is made, the aorta and vena cavae are cannulated and the patient placed on cardiopulmonary bypass. Right atriotomy is made and the defect and mitral valve are exposed. Closure of the mitral valve cleft with interrupted suture material and additional reparative procedures to address observed mitral valve abnormalities (for example, annuloplasty) should be undertaken. Then the atrial defect is closed using an autologous pericardial patch and rarely other prosthetic material (Dacron or Gore-Tex). Associated ostium secundum ASD or a patent foramen ovale should also be surgically closed at the same sitting.

3.4.4 Results

Results are generally good with a mortality rate less than 3%. The risk factors for poor results are severe mitral insufficiency, failure to thrive and congestive heart failure.

3.5 Prognosis

The prognosis is generally good. The actuarial survival at 20- and 40-year follow-up was 87% and 76% respectively for a large group of patients that had repair of ostium primum ASDs at Mayo Clinic (El-Najdawi et al 2000). The survival was better if the mitral valve repair was performed prior to 20 years of age. Repeat surgery, mostly to address mitral valve disease was required in 11% patients. Development of sub-aortic stenosis and heart block, requiring intervention occurs in a minority of patents during long-term follow-up.

4. Sinus venosus ASDs

Sinus venosus defects constitute 5 to 10% of all ASDs and the majority of defects are located in the posterior superior portion of the inter-atrial septum, often overriding the superior vena caval orifice. These defects are frequently associated with anomalous connection of the right upper pulmonary veins to the superior vena cava or right atrium near the cavo-atrial junction. The right pulmonary veins from the entire right lung may be connected anomalously. Rarely, the defect may be located in the inferior-posterior part of the atrial septum, overriding the inferior vena caval orifice. The dilatation of right heart structures is similar to that described in ostium secundum ASDs as are the clinical features. The ECG, in addition to the findings of rsR' pattern of the QRS complex shows somewhat superiorly oriented P wave vector (<30^0). Echocardiogram shows right ventricular volume overloading, similar to ostium secundum ASDs, but without an obvious ASD in the secondum position. Subcostal views may show the defect. Turbulence in the right upper pulmonary veins may also help suspect this diagnosis. The indications for intervention are also similar to those discussed in the ostium secundum ASD section. However, these defects are not amenable to transcatheter closure and surgical correction is the treatment of choice. Diversion of the anomalously connected right pulmonary vein(s) into the left atrium along with the closure of the ASD should be undertaken. This may involve constructing a tunnel with an autologous pericardial patch along with enlargement of superior vena cava.

5. Coronary sinus ASDs

These are rarest types of ASDs; these are defects in the inferior and anterior portion of the atrial septum at the expected location of the orifice of the coronary sinus. These defects are often associated with a persistent left superior vena cava and unroofing of the coronary sinus, a complex described as Raghib syndrome. The defect may be seen in association with asplenia syndrome. Dilatation of right heart structures and clinical features are similar to that described in ostium secundum ASD section. Echocardiogram is useful in the evaluation and diagnosis of this anomaly. Surgical correction with patch closure of the defect, leaving the entry of coronary sinus in the left atrium is the conventional method of approach (Lee and Sade 1979). These defects are not usually amenable to transcatheter closure. However, some, particularly small, defects may be amenable to transcatheter occlusion (Di Bernardo et al 2003)

6. Patent foramen ovale

To complete the discussion of defects in the atrial septum, a brief review of PFO is in order. The foramen ovale in the fetus is kept patent because of the mechanical effect of streaming of the inferior vena caval blood into the left atrium. At birth, a combination of increase in the left atrial pressure secondary to increased pulmonary venous return and decrease in the right atrial pressure due to eliminated placental return will result in apposition of the septum primum and septum secundum causing functional closure of the foramen ovale. Eventually anatomical closure occurs in most normal individuals.

Continued patency of the foramen ovale is critical in neonates with right heart obstructive lesions (tricuspid or pulmonary atresia) as well as left-sided obstructive lesions (hypoplastic left heart syndrome and mitral or aortic atresia) so as to allow an obligatory right-to-left or left-to-right shunt across the atrial septum, respectively. Similarly the patency of the foramen ovale is important in total anomalous pulmonary venous connection where all pulmonary and systemic venous returns come into the right atrium and consequently the systemic blood flow is entirely derived from right-to-left shunting across the PFO. In neonates with transposition of the great arteries (TGA), the circulation is parallel (instead of normal in-series circulation) and some inter-circulatory mixing is essential for survival; this is usually provided by the ASD/PFO. With any of the above scenarios the foramen ovale can become restrictive and may need enlargement either by transcatheter or surgical methodology (Rao 2007).

In patients with large patent ductus arteriosus (PDA) or ventricular septal defect (VSD), the pulmonary blood flow is markedly increased with consequent increase in the left atrial size; this left atrial enlargement may cause stretching of the patent foramen ovale resulting in an additional left-to-right atrial shunting. However, in clinical practice, the clinician needs to address the primary cardiac problem (PDA or VSD) and the PFO will either spontaneously resolve or become small so that it may not remain clinically significant.

The prevalence of PFO, based on autopsy studies is 27%; this incidence was 34% in the first thirty years of life which decreased to 25% in 30 to 80 year-olds which further decreased to 20% in 80 to 100-year-olds (Hagen 1984). Similar prevalence was observed by TEE examinations. Consequently the PFO should be considered a normal variant. However, some these PFOs are considered to be the seat of right to left shunt causing paradoxical embolism and cerebrovascular accidents (Lechat et al 1988, Webster et al 1988, Ende et al 1996, Windecker and Meier 2003) and hypoxemia as seen in platypnea-orthodeoxia syndrome (Waight et al 2000, Rao et al 2001). Right to left shunt thru' PFO can also occur in patients who were previously treated for complex congenital cardiac anomalies (Rao et al 1997), including Fontan fenestrations as well as in patients who had right ventricular infarction (Bassi et al 2005). Decompression (Caisson's) illness (Wilmshurst et al 1996, Walsh et al 1999, Wilmshurst et al 2000) and migrane (Wilmshurst et al 2000) have also been attributed to right to left shunt across PFO. There is varying degrees of evidence regarding the benefits of transcatheter occlusion of PFOs in above described conditions; some of these issues are addressed in later chapters of this book.

7. Summary and conclusions

In this review, the clinical features and management of ASDs are discussed. Four types of defects namely, ostium secondum, ostium primum, sinus venosus and coronar sinus ASDs are included. Patients with small defects, especially in childhood, are usually asymptomatic while moderate to large defects in infancy, though rarely, may present with symptoms.

Physical findings include hyperdynamic precordium, widely split and fixed second heart sound, ejection systolic murmur at the left upper sternal border and a mid-diastolic flow rumble at the left lower sternal border. Clinical diagnosis is not usually difficult and the diagnosis can be confirmed and quantified by non-invasive echocardiographic studies. Whereas surgical intervention was used in the past, transcatheter methods are currently used for closure of ostium secondum ASDs. Surgical correction is usually necessary for the other three types of defects.

PFO is present in nearly one third of normal population and is likely to be a normal variant. In the presence of some structural abnormalities of the heart, their presence may facilitate intra-cardiac shunt to allow appropriate egress and/or mixing of blood flow. PFOs, presumed to be the seat of paradoxical embolism resulting in stroke/transient ischemic attacks deserve special consideration. Hypoxemia in post-surgical residual defects including Fontan fenestrations and right ventricular infarction may be secondary to right to left shunt across PFO. Other problems such as migraine, Caisson's disease and platypnea-orthodexia syndrome are also attributed to shunts across PFO. Evidence for benefit of transcatheter occlusion of these PFOs is variable.

8. References

[1] Bassi, S.; Amersey. R.; Andrews, R. (2005) Right ventricular infarction complicated by right to left shunting through an atrial septal defect: successful treatment with an Amplatzer septal occluder, *Heart,* Vol. 91, No. 4, pp. e28.

[2] Carcagnì, A.; Presbitero, P. (2004) New echocardiographic diameter for Amplatzer sizing in adult patients with secundum atrial septal defect: preliminary results, *Catheter Cardiovasc Interv,* Vol. 62, No. 3, pp. 409-414.

[3] Chopra, PS.; Rao, PS. (2000) History of development of atrial septal occlusion devices, *Current Intervent Cardiol Reports,* Vol. 2, No. 1, pp. 63-69.

[4] Di Bernardo, S.; Fasnacht, M,; Berger, F. (2003)Transcatheter closure of a coronary sinus defect with an Amplatzer septal occluder. *Catheter Cardiovasc Interv,* Vol. 60, No. 2, pp.287-290.

[5] El-Najdawi, E.; Driscoll, D.; Puga, F.; et al. (2000) Operation for partial atrioventricular septal defect: A 40-year review, *J Thorac Cardiovsc Surg,* Vol. 119, No. 5, pp. 880-889.

[6] Ende, DJ. ; Chopra, PS. ; Rao, PS. (1996) Transcatheter closure of atrial septal defect or patent foramen ovale with the buttoned device for prevention of recurrence of paradoxic embolism, *Am J Cardiol,* Vol. 78, No. 2, pp. 233-236.

[7] Hagen, PT.; Scholz, DG.; Edwards, WD. (1984) Incidence and size of patent foramen ovale during the first 10 decades of life: an autopsy study of 965 normal hearts. Mayo Clin Proc, Vol . 59, No. 1, pp. 17-20.

[8] Hamdan, MA. ; Cao, Q. ; Hijazi, ZM. (2003) Amplatzer septal occluder, In: *Catheter Based Devices for Treatment of Noncoronary Cardiovascular Disease in Adults and Children,* P.S. Rao, M.J. Kern. (Eds.): 51-59, Lippincott, Williams & Wilkins, Philadelphia, PA, USA

[9] Jones, TK.; Latson, LA. ; Zahn, E, ; et al. (2007) Multicenter Pivotal Study of the HELEX Septal Occluder Investigators. Results of the U.S. multicenter pivotal study of the HELEX septal occluder for percutaneous closure of secundum atrial septal defects, *J Am Coll Cardiol,* Vol. 49, No. 22 , pp. 2215-2221

[10] Lee, ME.; Sade, RM. (1979) Coronary sinus septal defect: surgical considerations, *J Thorac Cardiovasc Surg*, Vol 78, No. 4, pp. 563-569.

[11] Latson, LA.; Wilson, N.; Zahn, EM. (2003) Helex setal occluder. In: *Catheter Based Devices for Treatment of Noncoronary Cardiovascular Disease in Adults and Children*, P.S. Rao, M.J. Kern. (Eds.): 71-78, Lippincott, Williams & Wilkins, Philadelphia, PA, USA

[12] Lechat, P.; Mas, JL.; Lascault, G.; et al. (1988) Prevalence of patent foramen ovale in patients with stroke. N Engl J Med. Vol. 318, No. 18, pp. 1148-1152.

[13] Murphy, JG.; Gersh, BJ.; McGoon, MD.; et al. (1990) Long-term outcome after surgical repair of isolated atrial septal defect. *New Engl J Med*, Vol. 323, No. 24, pp. 1645-1650.

[14] Nagm, AM.; Rao, PS. (2004) Percutaneous occlusion of complex atrial septal defects. *J Invasive Cardiol*, Vol. 16, No. 3, pp. 123-125.

[15] Rao, PS. (1998) Transcatheter closure of atrial septal defects: Are we there yet? (editorial). *J Am Coll Cardiol*, Vol. 31, No. 5, pp. 1117-1119.

[16] Rao, PS. (2000) Summary and comparison of atrial septal closure devices. *Current Intervent Cardiol Reports*, Vol. 2, No. 4, pp. 367-376.

[17] Rao, PS. (2003) History of atrial septal occlusion devices. In: *Catheter Based Devices for Treatment of Noncoronary Cardiovascular Disease in Adults and Children*, P.S. Rao, M.J. Kern. (Eds.): 1-9, Lippincott, Williams & Wilkins, Philadelphia, PA, USA

[18] Rao, PS. (2003) Comparative summary of atrial septal defect occlusion devices. In: *Catheter Based Devices for Treatment of Noncoronary Cardiovascular Disease in Adults and Children*, P.S. Rao, M.J. Kern. (Eds.): 91-101, Lippincott, Williams & Wilkins, Philadelphia, PA, USA

[19] Rao, PS. (2007) Role of Interventional Cardiology In Neonates: Part I. Non-Surgical Atrial Septostomy. *Congenital Cardiol Today*, Vol. 5, No. 12, pp. 1-12.

[20] Rao, PS.; Awa, S.; Linde, LM. (1973) Role of Kinetic Energy in Pulmonary Valvar Pressure Gradients. *Circulation* Vol. 48, No. 1, pp. 65-73.

[21] Rao, PS.; Berger, F., Rey, C.; Haddad, J.; et al. (2000) Results of Transvenous Occlusion of Secundum Atrial Septal Defects with 4th Generation Buttoned Device: Comparison with 1st, 2nd and 3rd Generation Devices. *J Am Coll Cardiol*, Vol. 36, No. 2, pp. 583-592

[22] Rao, PS.; Sideris, EB. (2001) Centering-on-demand Buttoned Device: Its Role in Transcatheter Occlusion of Atrial Septal Defects, *J Intervent Cardiol*, Vol. 14, No. 1, pp. 81-89.

[23] Rao, PS.; Sideris, EB.; Hausdorf G.; et al. (1994) International Experience with Secundum Atrial Septal Defect Occlusion by The Buttoned Device, *Am Heart J*, Vol. 128, No. 5, pp. 1022-1035.

[24] Rao, PS.; Wilson, AD.; Levy, JM.; Chopra, PS. (1992) Role of "Buttoned" Double-disk Device in the Management of Atrial Septal Defects, *Am Heart J*, Vol. 123, No. 1, pp. 191-200.

[25] Rao, PS.; Chandar, JS.; Sideris, EB. (1997) Role of inverted buttoned device in transcatheter occlusion of atrial septal defect or patent foramen ovale with right-to-left shunting associated with previously operated complex congenital cardiac anomalies, *Am J Cardiol*, Vol. 80, No. 7, pp. 914-921.

[26] Rao PS, Palacios IF, Bach RG, et al. (2001) Platypnea-orthodeoxia syndrome: management by transcatheter buttoned device implantation, *Cathet Cardiovasc Intervent,* Vol. 54, No. 1, pp. 77-82.

[27] Waight, DJ.; Cao, QL.; Hijazi, ZM. (2000) Closure of patent foramen ovale in patients with orthodeoxia-platypnea using the amplatzer devices, *Catheter Cardiovasc Interv,* Vol. 50, No. 2, pp.195-198.

[28] Walsh, KP.; Wilmshurst, PT.; Morrison WL. (1999) Transcatheter closure of patent foramen ovale using the Amplatzer septal occluder to prevent recurrence of neurological decompression illness in divers, *Heart,* Vol. 81, No. 3, pp. 257-261.

[29] Webster MW, Chancellor AM, Smith HJ, et al. (1988) Patent foramen ovale in young stroke patients, *Lancet,* Vol. 2, No. 8601, pp. 11-12.

[30] Wilmshurst P, Nightingale S, Walsh KP et al. (2000) Effect on migraine of closure cardiac right-to-left shunts to prevent recurrence of decompression illness, stroke or for haemodynamic reasons, *Lancet,* Vol. 356, No. 9242, pp. 1648-1651.

[31] Wilmshurst P, Walsh K, Morrison WL. (1996) Transcatheter occlusion of foramen ovale with a buttoned device after neurological decompression illness in professional divers, *Lancet,* Vol. 348, No. 9029, pp. 752-753.

[32] Windecker S, Meier B. (2003) Percutaneous closure of patent foramen ovale in patients with presumed paradoxical embolism. In: *Catheter Based Devices for Treatment of Noncoronary Cardiovascular Disease in Adults and Children,* P.S. Rao, M.J. Kern. (Eds.): 111-118, Lippincott, Williams & Wilkins, Philadelphia, PA, USA

2

Pregnancy Issues in Women with Atrial Septal Defect

Duraisamy Balaguru
University of Texas-Houston Medical School, USA

1. Introduction

Success of surgical repair of congenital heart defects in the past five decades has enabled survival into adulthood. Women born with congenital heart diseases reach child-bearing age with or without surgical repair of those lesions. Specifically, atrial septal defect (ASD) is a non-lethal, acyanotic lesion in which survival into adulthood with or without surgery is common place. Types of ASD and hemodynamics have been discussed elsewhere in this book. Briefly, ASD causes left to right shunting leading to right atrial and right ventricular enlargement and increased pulmonary blood flow. Heart failure is uncommon before 4th decade. Mild pulmonary arterial hypertension may occur with advancing age. However, Eisenmenger's syndrome is rare.

Presence of ASD may be diagnosed for the first time during adulthood - probably during pregnancy when an asymptomatic murmur is evaluated using echocardiography. Pregnancy causes cardiovascular changes due to fetal demand for oxygen and nutrition and due to effect of maternal hormones on blood volume and hematocrit. In this chapter, effects of these cardiovascular changes on ASD hemodynamics and effect of ASD on the pregnancy will be discussed. Management strategies will be reviewed.

2. Physiologic changes during pregnancy

2.1 Cardiovascular changes

Physiologic demands of pregnancy lead to significant changes in cardiovascular system during pregnancy, labor and postpartum (Strong et al. 1992). Cardiac output increases constantly in the first 30 weeks of pregnancy reaching ~140% of the pre-gestational level. After 30 weeks, the increase is minimal. Initially, stroke volume increases more than the heart rate. In later part of pregnancy, heart rate increases. There is a 10-fold increase in blood flow to placenta and uterus during pregnancy. Since placenta offers very low vascular resistance, maternal systemic vascular resistance decreases. A reduction in left ventricular afterload occurs (Metcalfe & Ueland 1974). A corresponding increase in cardiac output occurs during the same period, keeping blood pressure stable in spite of the reduction in afterload.

Overall, circulatory changes can be summarized as follows: Increase in stroke volume by 18-25% with heart rate increase by 20%. Net effect of this is a 30-50% increase in cardiac output.

There is increased extraction of oxygen by the placenta leading to increase in arterio-venous difference of oxygen content. Both systemic and pulmonary vascular resistance decrease. However, the reduction in systemic vascular resistance is higher leading to decrease in left to right shunting across ASD. Systemic blood pressure shows a reduction in both systolic and diastolic pressure with a higher reduction in diastolic pressure, thus leading to a wide pulse pressure. (Perloff, JK et al.1992).

2.2 Respiratory changes

Concurrent to cardiovascular changes, changes occur in the respiratory system as well. There is a 45% increase in minute ventilation and 20% increase in oxygen consumption. There is a mild increase in respiratory rate. Functional residual capacity increases by approximately 40% (Perloff, JK et al. 1992).

2.3 Hematologic changes

Due to hormonal changes, blood volume increases to about 150% of the pre-gestational value (Figure 1). This is accomplished by increase in plasma volume out of proportion to the increase in red cell mass. Therefore, "physiologic" anemia occurs which in turn imposes a hyperdynamic circulatory state (Figure 1).

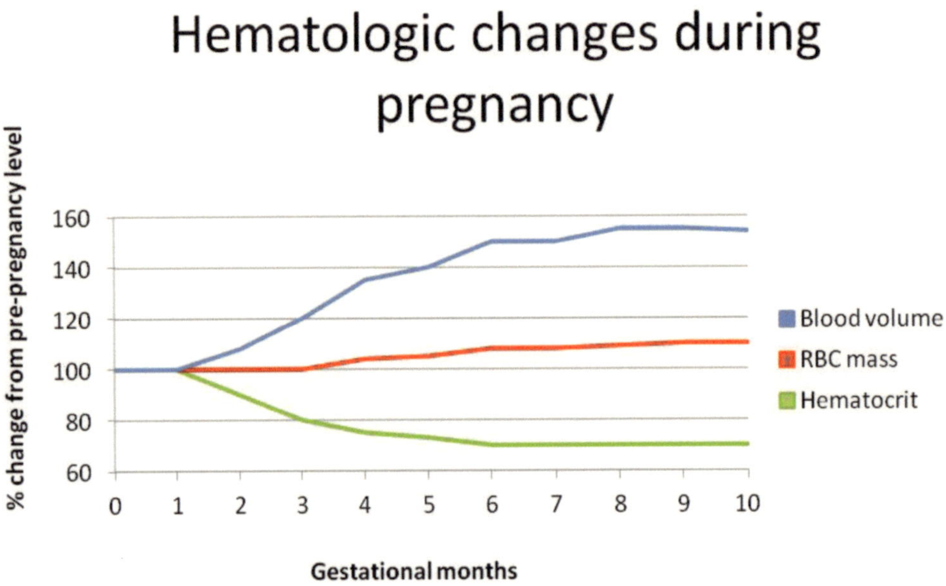

Fig. 1. Hematologic changes during pregnancy. Changes in blood volume, red cell mass (RBC mass) and hematocrit occur during pregnancy. RBC mass increases only approximately 110% while blood volume increases by approximately 150% resulting in "physiologic" anemia of pregnancy. (Figure adapted from Strong et al. 1992).

Greatest demand on the cardiovascular system occurs after 30 weeks of gestation. This is usually tolerated well in woman with normal heart or mild heart disease before conception (New York Heart Association Functional Class I and II) because the demand increases gradually. Increasing fetal demand of oxygen is met with increasing placental blood flow and slight increase in maternal hyperventilation in late pregnancy (Pitkin et al. 1990).

2.4 Changes in last trimester and labor

During the last trimester, enlarging uterus compresses the inferior vena cava (IVC) especially in supine posture resulting in two effects. One, decrease in venous return leading to decrease in cardiac output in supine posture. Second, predisposition to deep vein thrombosis in lower part of the body by creating sluggish circulation. (Metcalfe 1978).

During labor, significant changes occur in a short period of time. In first stage of labor, uterine contractions lead to compression of IVC and decrease in venous capacitances and increase in systemic vascular resistance. This leads to reduction in cardiac output during uterine contractions. However, when the uterus relaxes the cardiac output increases back to pre-contraction levels. In second stage of labor, cardiac output increases significantly due to vigorous expulsive effort. (Ueland & Metcalfe 1975).

After delivery, removal of placenta leads to increase in systemic vascular resistance. Blood loss during labor is a stress on the heart. Equally important is the fact that several hormonal stimuli that occur during pregnancy are receding during postpartum, leading to return of blood volume, hematocrit and cardiac output to pre-conception levels.

3. Effect of pregnancy on ASD

Hemodynamic changes outlined above will affect the hemodynamics of ASD. In a study of 54 pregnant women with ASD, an increase in right atrial and right ventricular size was found, more than the control group of pregnant women who did not have any heart defect. Indirect parameters of right ventricular strain were worse and estimated proportion of pulmonary blood flow to systemic blood flow was lower. There was a higher incidence of supraventricular tachycardia during pregnancy in women with ASD. (Peisiewicz et al. 2004).

Higher incidence of thromboembolism during pregnancy due to venous stasis in the lower part of the body and hypercoagulable state due to high progesterone level was detected. Increased respiratory effort during pregnancy from hemodynamic changes and anemia, and straining during parturition increase the chances of paradoxical embolism. These risks have been reported in several cases in the literature and raise the issue of whether closure of ASD during pregnancy is indicated.

4. Effect of ASD on pregnancy

Asymptomatic ASD without functional compromise (NYHA Class I and II) usually have no effect on pregnancy. However, if there is pre-existing heart failure, there is decrease in uterine blood flow leading to compromised fetal growth (reflected in incidence of small for gestation age babies) and viability. In a review that consolidated outcome of 123 pregnancies in women with ASD, 1 arrhytmic event, no heart failure events, 2 cardiovascular events and 1 endocarditis were reported. In this study, incidence of these reported events were less than what is expected for healthy women. Similarly, incidence of adverse neonatal events was also low including small for premature birth, small for gestational age and neonatal mortality (Drenthem et al. 2007).

5. Risk of inheritance of ASD in the offspring

If there is a recognizable genetic syndrome in the mother associated with ASD, the inheritance pattern of such syndrome will dictate the risk of congenital heart disease in the fetus. In the absence of such genetic syndrome in the mother, incidence of congenital heart disease is 2-4% if mother has congenital heart disease which is higher than 0.6 – 0.8% incidence in general population. In a Danish study of 1.7 million persons, a recurrence risk of 7.1 in first-degree relatives of individuals with congenital heart disease. (Oyen et al. 2009). Another European study from Netherland, reported an occurrence of ASD in 2.4% of the offspring in a cohort of 291 pregnancies in women with ASD. (Drenthen et al. 2007)

6. Management of pregnancy with ASD

Management pregnancy in women with ASD depends on whether the ASD was diagnosed prior to pregnancy, size of ASD and pre-existing cardiac issues related to ASD such as chamber enlargement, heart failure, arrhythmia and pulmonary artery hypertension. In general, uncomplicated ASD need not be treated during pregnancy.

6.1 Diagnosis known before pregnancy

If the diagnosis of ASD were known prior to pregnancy and ASD is large associated with hemodynamically-significant shunt, associated with moderate or severe chamber enlargement, a potential for supraventricular tachycardia and thromboembolic events during pregnancy, labor or postpartum. Therefore, the patient should have ASD closed prior to planned-pregnancy. Current practice is to electively close asymptomatic, but significant size ASDs prior to child-bearing years. Transcatheter or surgical technique should be applied based on the location and size of ASD and presence of adequate rim of tissue around the ASD suitable for transcatheter device placement. If unsuitable for transcatheter closure, surgical repair is sought.

6.2 ASD diagnosed during pregnancy

6.2.1 Medical management

ASD does not always require surgical or transcatheter closure. If the pregnant woman is asymptomatic (NYHA Functional Class I and II) without heart failure, atrial arrhythmia or pulmonary hypertension or history of stroke, an expectant management of ASD during pregnancy is acceptable. However, if any of the above stated risk factors exist, ASD may need to be closed during pregnancy. Indications for intervention (surgical or transcatheter options) include severe hemodynamic compromise, NYHA class > II, recurrent stroke prior to or during pregnancy, etc. This usually constitutes a small number of patients. Medical treatment of arrhythmia may be necessary during pregnancy.

6.2.2 Transcatheter closure of ASD during pregnancy

Indication for treatment of ASD during pregnancy includes high risk of recurrent stroke, high risk for taking anticoagulation throughout pregnancy such as intracranial hemorrhage, prior intolerance to anticoagulation with complicating bleeding, thrombocytopenia, hypertension, preeclampsia or other system impairment such as renal or liver dysfunction.

Several precautions are taken if such procedure is required. Radiation of the fetus and its teratogenic effect are an important consideration during transcatheter therapy for ASD. First trimester irradiation will be associated with higher incidence of fetal malformation. Therefore, catheterization is performed in second trimester (13-28 weeks). Use of long venous sheath avoids direct radiation exposure and reduces radiation dose to pelvic area. Use of intracardiac echocardiography for balloon sizing and guidance of device deployment greatly reduces overall radiation exposure to the mother as well as the fetus. (Orchard et al. 2011) (Schrale et al. 2007). General anesthesia may be avoided by use of local anesthesia with conscious sedation for the catheterization procedure.

6.2.3 Surgical closure of ASD during pregnancy

Indication for surgical closure of ASD is rare. However, if the abovementioned indications for ASD closure exist and the ASD is unsuitable for transcatheter closure, surgical closure of ASD is indicated. Following precautions are suggested based on several observations. Ideal period for open heart surgery during pregnancy is second trimester (13 - 28 weeks) in order to avoid any fetal malformations (first trimester) and to avoid preterm labor, unfavorable maternal hemodynamics and increased maternal mortality (third trimester). During surgery, fetal bradycardia at the start of cardiopulmonary bypass may be avoided by infusion of high-concentration glucose to provide energy for fetus and intraoperative monitoring of fetal well being with cardiotachometer and fetal echocardiogram. During cardiopulmonary bypass, high-flow and high mean arterial pressure (60 mmHg), hyperoxygenation and maintenance of high hematocrit (> 25%) are advised. (Arnoni et al. 2003).

7. Outcome

A study compared pregnancy outcome in women who have had surgical repair of ASD before conception with women who have not had repair. 60 women (115 pregnancies) had surgery for ASD while 20 women (48 pregnancies) had unrepaired ASD. Incidence of still births, recurrence of congenital heart defect in the offspring or long term cardiac complications were similar in both groups. However, incidence of miscarriage, preterm delivery and cardiac symptoms during pregnancy were higher in women who had unrepaired ASD. (Actis Dato et al. 1998).

Drenthen et al. (2007) reported 0.8% incidence of arrhythmias, no cases of heart failure during pregnancy, 5% occurrence of thromboembolic events in women with ASD. Figure 2 provides the perspective of risk to the offspring in women with ASD compared with various congenital heart diseases. While outcome of pregnancy relatively better with ASD compared to other congenital heart diseases, a certain incidence of complications have been reported including preterm delivery (6%), small for gestational age at birth (2%), fetal mortality (2.4%), perinatal mortality (1.7%) and recurrence of heart disease (2%). (Drenthen et al. 2007)

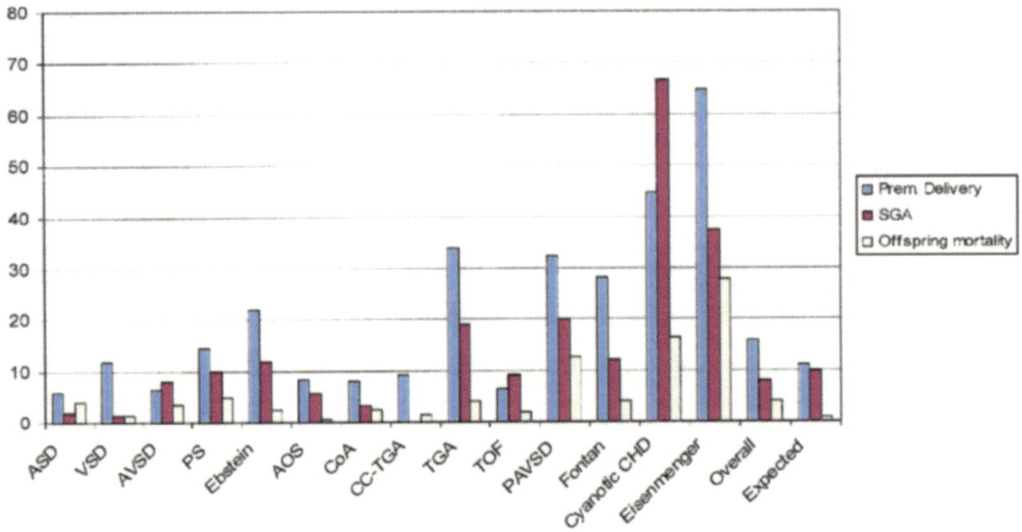

Fig. 2. Risk to the offspring from pregnancy in women with ASD compared to women with other congenital heart diseases. (Reproduced with permission. Drenthen et al 2007).

8. Contraception

Pregnancy is not contraindicated in women with ASD. However, there may be social and other clinical circumstances that may require delaying ASD closure and therefore, the pregnancy. In such circumstances, conception may be used. Since ASD is an acyanotic heart disease, there are more options compared to women with cyanotic heart disease. Barrier methods and intrauterine devices may be used. When these devices are inserted or removed, endocarditis prophylaxis is not indicated in patients with ASD. Though not crucial, progesterone-only pills have lesser incidence of thromboembolism compared to combination pills of estrogen and progesterone. However, progesterone-only pills may cause irregular bleeding especially in the first month of use. Efficacy of progesterone-only pills is slightly lower than combined contraceptive pills. Similarly, the morning-after pills are also safe and effective for women with heart disease. There are injectable forms of long-acting contraceptives available. From cardiac point of view, permanent methods of sterilization such as tubal ligation or vasectomy for the partner are unwarranted in cases with ASD.

9. Conclusion

Pregnancy in women without heart disease has its own risks. Women with ASD who are asymptomatic, NYHA Class I or II are likely to have uneventful pregnancy. The ASD may be closed either surgically or by transcatheter technique if found suitable. For high risk patients, treatment of ASD during pregnancy may be undertaken. Second trimester is considered suitable for either transcatheter or surgical repair of ASD. Radiation dose is minimized by using intracardiac echocardiogram and modifications of the catheter procedure. Similarly, precautions are taken during open heart surgery should surgical repair were necessary. However, such need for closure of ASD during pregnancy should be rare and if possible avoided.

10. References

Actis Dato GM, Rinaudo P, Revelli A, et al. (1998). Atrial septal defect and pregnancy: a retrospective analysis of obstetrical outcome before and after surgical correction. Minerva Cardioangiol. 46:63-68.

Arnoni, RT, Arnoni, AS, Bonini, RC, et al. (2003) Risk factors associated with cardiac surgery during pregnancy. 76:1605-8.

Drenthen, W., Peiper, P.G., Roos-Hesselink, J.W. et al. (2007). Outcome of pregnancy in women with congenital heart disease. J Am Coll Cardiol 49:2303-2311.

Metcalfe, J. (1978). The heart in pregnancy: a guide to practical considerations. Hospital Medicine 9:95.

Metcalfe, J., Ueland, K. (1974). Maternal cardiovascular adjustments in pregnancy. Cardiovasc Dis 7:363-374.

Orchard EA, Wilson N, Ormerod OJ. (2011). Device closure of atrial septal defect during pregnancy for recurrent cerebrovascular accidents. Int J Cardiol 148:240-241.

Oyen, N., Poulsen, G., Boyd, H.A., et al. (2009). Recurrence of congenital heart defects in families. Circulation 2009;120:295-301.

Peisiewicz, W, Goch, A. Blinikowski, Z, et al. (2004). Changes in the cardiovascular system during pregnancy in women with secumdum atrial septal defect. Kardiol Pol. 60:218-228.

Perloff, JK, Koos, BJ. (1992) Pregnancy and congenital heart disease In: *Congenital Heart Disease in Adults,* Perloff, JK & Childs, JS. pp.(144-164) Saunders. Philadelphia, PA.

Pitkin, RM, Perloff, JK, Koos, BJ, Beall, MH. (1990) Pregnancy and congenital heart disease. Annals of Internal Medicine 112:445-454.

Schrale RG, Ormerod J, Ormerod OJ. (2007). Percutaneous device closure of the patent foramen ovale during pregnancy. Catheter Cardiovasc Interv 69:579 583.

Strong, W. et al. (1992). Sexuality, contraception and pregnancy in patients with cyanotic congenital heart disease with special reference to tricuspid atresia In: *Tricuspid Atresia*, Rao, P.S. pp.415-427. Futura Publishing Company, Inc., ISBN No. 0-87993-5189, Mount Kisco, NY.

Ueland, K., Metcalfe, J. (1975). Circulatory changes during pregnancy. Clin Obstet Gynecol 18:41-50.

Section 2

Natural History

3

Prevalence of Secundum Atrial Septal Defect and Associated Findings

Mark D. Reller
Oregon Health & Science University, USA

1. Introduction

The goal of this chapter is to review data regarding the *current* prevalence estimates for secundum type atrial septal defect (ASD) and to give the reader a sense as to how these prevalence data compare relative to other common cardiac defects. This chapter will also review the current understanding of cardiac and non-cardiac findings known to be associated with secundum ASD. It is recognized that the prevalence estimates of cardiac defects have been impacted by the routine utilization of color flow Doppler-echocardiography in current clinical practice. This is particularly true for certain cardiac anomalies such as secundum ASD that frequently occur in asymptomatic infants and children. Several studies have indeed documented a significant increase in the apparent prevalence of congenital heart defects in general and specifically for certain common phenotypes including secundum ASD (Hoffman & Kaplan, 2002; Wren et al., 2000; Correa et al., 2007). Further, these studies have concluded that much of these increases are likely secondary to better ascertainment in recent years. This chapter will review the most recent estimates of the prevalence of secundum ASD using information obtained from a population-based surveillance system using strict definitions of what constitutes a secundum ASD. This chapter will also review a detailed list of what is presently known about the associated findings and potential risk factors for the development of secundum ASD.

2. Definition of what constitutes a secundum ASD

One of the difficulties recognized with the utilization of standard trans-thoracic color-Doppler echocardiography is the inability to differentiate a small secundum ASD from the physiologic communication (the patent foramen ovale) seen in most newborn infants. In other words, deciding what constitutes a "true" ASD has obvious implications for making accurate estimates of prevalence. In a recently revised heart classification system, the diagnosis of secundum ASD was made only when the atrial defect is greater than or equal to 4 mm in diameter (Riehle-Colarusso et al., 2007). If the specific size of the defect is not indicated in the imaging study, the diagnosis of ASD can also be made in the presence of documented right heart enlargement. In clinical practice, one can sometimes detect a flap associated with patent foramen ovale even in defects larger than 4 mm. However, as this finding is not reliably reported, the utilization of the 4 mm size requirement for secundum ASD was chosen. While admittedly arbitrary, this size is based on previous published studies showing that most (if not all) defects less than this size close spontaneously and are therefore not considered anatomic atrial defects (Ghisla et al., 1995; Radzik et al., 1993). The prevalence data that are reported for secundum ASD in this chapter utilized this strict size cutoff. Investigations that do not make this distinction between small ASD and patent foramen ovale would be expected to give much higher estimates for the prevalence of secundum ASD.

It is well recognized that secundum ASD commonly occurs with other congenital cardiac defects. When it occurs with other presumed "independent" heart defects (such as with ventricular septal defects), most investigators, when assessing prevalence, would count ASD as a distinct cardiac defect. However, when a secundum ASD occurs as an *obligatory* shunt (such as with the diagnoses of tricuspid and pulmonary atresia, transposition of the great arteries, complex single ventricle with mitral atresia, or hypoplastic left heart syndrome), it is typically *not* counted as a distinct cardiac defect. The prevalence data reported in this chapter were made using these same distinctions.

3. Background and methods

One challenge in assessing differences in prevalence of congenital cardiac defects across population groups and over time has been the variation in nomenclature and classification systems that have been utilized. The prevalence data reviewed in this chapter were obtained utilizing the Metropolitan Atlanta Congenital Defects Program (MACDP) using data that were analyzed for births that occurred between 1998 and 2005 (the most recent time-frame studied) (Reller et al., 2008). A major strength of the MACDP is that it is a population-based surveillance system that includes structural birth defects, chromosomal abnormalities, and clinical syndromes. It was established in 1967 by the Centers for Disease Control and Prevention (CDC), Emory University, and the Georgia Mental Health Institute (Correa et al., 2007). This program has conducted surveillance for birth defects among live born and stillborn infants greater than 20 weeks gestation born to residents of the 5 central counties of metropolitan Atlanta through the use of active case-finding methods. While many of the cardiac defects in MACDP are diagnosed in infancy, cases can be ascertained *up to 6 years of age*. The MACDP recently completed a re-classification of all heart defects in its database (Riehle-Colarusso et al., 2007). All cases underwent a detailed review by pediatric cardiologists to classify congenital heart defects according to standard nomenclature used by the Society of Thoracic Surgeons congenital heart surgery database (Jacobs et al., 2004).

4. Prevalence of secundum ASD

Prevalence estimates are reported per 10,000 live births with the numerators representing the number of *infants* with secundum ASD (or any other cardiac defect) per 10,000 live births. The current overall prevalence of congenital heart defects is estimated to be 81.4 infants per 10,000 births (~0.8% of live births). The prevalence of secundum ASD is estimated to be 10.3 per 10,000 births. As a frame of reference, the most common cardiac defect is muscular ventricular septal defect (VSD) with a prevalence of 27.5 per 10,000 live births. It is noteworthy that the prevalence of secundum ASD is comparable to peri-membranous VSD (prevalence of 10.6 per 10,000 live births) and greater than any other specific cardiac defect (Reller et al., 2008). Based on current prevalence data, secundum ASD is the third most common cardiac defect, and together with muscular and peri-membranous VSD, account for slightly more than half of all recognized cardiac defects.

Secundum ASD is by far the most common of the atrial septal defects, accounting for greater than 80% of all atrial defects where the specific sub-type is identified. Secundum ASD is ~ 6 times more common than the ostium primum type ASD (1.7 per 10,000 live births) and ~ 25 times more common than the sinus venosus atrial septal defect (0.4 per 10,000 live births) (Reller et al., 2008).

Last, it is recognized in clinical practice that many individuals with ASD are diagnosed later in life and indeed, are the most common un-diagnosed congenital cardiac defect presenting in adult congenital cardiology clinics (Rosas et al., 2004). Thus, while the prevalence data obtained from the MACDP database are the most current available, it is clear that these data (diagnosed in infants and children), are under-estimates of the "true" prevalence of secundum ASD.

5. Associations and risk factors

The cause(s) of secundum ASD, as is true for most congenital heart defects, remain largely unknown. Nonetheless, there are clearly recognized associations between secundum ASD and other cardiac and non-cardiac findings that are worth reviewing and may ultimately help to elucidate an etiology for at least some of the causes for secundum ASD. These associations are discussed in the paragraphs that follow.

5.1 Associations with other cardiac defects

Several investigations have documented the association of secundum ASD with peri-membranous VSD as well as with valvular pulmonary stenosis (Botto et al., 2007). The relative frequency and non-randomness of these associations suggest that they may have specific risk factor profiles. Indeed, there is some suggestion that the combination of secundum ASD and peri-membranous VSD *within families* may occur in greater frequency in the setting of the NKX2-5 genotype (Schott et al., 1998).

5.2 Genetic syndromes

Infants with secundum ASD are more likely to have a positive family history of congenital heart disease than most other cardiac defects (Ferencz et al., 1997). The finding of a positive family history obviously suggests the possibility of genetic causation(s) yet to be determined. There are several recognized genetic syndromes that have been shown to be associated with secundum ASD. While Trisomy 21 is more commonly associated with the finding of partial or complete atrio-ventricular septal defects, infants with Down syndrome also have an increased risk for isolated secundum ASD as well (Ferencz et al., 1997; Boldt et al., 2002). It is generally recognized that secundum ASD is also seen in greater frequency with the chromosomal anomalies Trisomy 13 and 18.

Other recognized genetic syndromes associated with an increased risk of secundum ASD include the Holt-Oram syndrome, where the association of radial limb anomalies and cardiac defects, primarily secundum ASD, is seen in at least half of affected individuals (Basson et al., 1994). Secundum ASD is also seen with chromosome 22q11 deletion in association with DiGeorge syndrome and velo-cardio-facial syndrome (Borgman et al., 1999). Secundum ASD, occurring either in isolation, or in conjunction with pulmonary stenosis, is associated with Noonan syndrome (Mendez and Opitz, 1985). The NKX2-5 gene defect has been shown to be associated with *familial causes* of either isolated secundum ASD, or in combination with other cardiac defects, and with heart rhythm conduction anomalies (Schott et al., 1998; Benson et al., 1999).

5.3 Female gender

The association with female gender has long been recognized. In the current prevalence estimates, secundum ASD was significantly more common in girls (58.6%) than boys. (Reller et al., 2008). In the Baltimore-Washington Infant Study, 65.3% of children with secundum ASD were girls (Ferencz et al., 1997).

5.4 Non-cardiac malformations and pregnancy exposures/teratogens

Certain common non-cardiac malformations such as cleft palate are associated with an increased incidence of secundum ASD (Ferencz et al., 1997). Some of these infants will have chromosome 22q11 deletion, as noted above. Secundum ASD is the most common congenital cardiac defect associated with a constellation of non-cardiac anomalies recognized as the VACTERL (Vertebral anomalies, Anal atresia, Cardiac defects, Tracheal anomalies, Esophageal atresia, Renal anomalies, and Limb anomalies) association (Ferencz et al., 1997).

In addition, certain pregnancy exposures have been shown to be associated with secundum ASD and include maternal alcohol ingestion (fetal alcohol syndrome) (Mone et al., 2004). Exposure to certain viral infections such as cytomegalovirus (CMV) and rubella infections during pregnancy are also associated with an increased risk for secundum ASD (Ferencz et al., 1997). Last, the presence of maternal diabetes including gestational diabetes is associated with an increased risk of cardiac defects including secundum ASD (Ferencz et al., 1997; Loffredo al., 2001).

5.5 Other pregnancy and pre-pregnancy-related "risk factors"

As a group, infants with secundum ASD, compared to live-born infants in the general population, are significantly more likely to be born at a lower gestational age and have significantly lower birth weight (Reller et al., 2008; Ferencz et al., 1997). Further, infants with secundum ASD are more likely to be small for gestational age irrespective of their gestational age at delivery. Last, infants with secundum ASD (relative to infants in the general population), are more likely to be born of mothers of increased maternal age and are significantly more likely to be the product of a multiple gestation pregnancy (Reller et al., 2008; Mastroiacovo et al., 1999).

The cause(s) of the association of secundum ASD with low gestational age and low birth weight is unclear at the current time. One possibility is that ASD might somehow impair normal fetal growth. Another possibility is that both altered fetal growth and secundum ASD represent co-outcomes of an associated causal risk factor. Clearly, more investigation is necessary.

Current data indicate that both older maternal age and multiple-gestation pregnancy are associated with secundum ASD. In addition, the association with older maternal age appears to be independent of the increased risk of genetic syndromes that occurs with older maternal age (Reller et al., 2008). It is recognized that older maternal age is more likely to be associated with the use of assisted reproductive technology, which is a strong risk factor for multiple gestation pregnancy. Thus, these findings of maternal age and multiple-gestation pregnancy may be inter-related. It is noteworthy that over the past 4 decades, one important demographic change has occurred in our society. In 1968, roughly 16% of mothers at the time of delivery were 30 years old or older compared with 42% in 2005 (Correa et al., 2007). During this same timeframe, the number of multiple-gestation pregnancies also nearly doubled from 1.8% to 3.4%.

Last, recent epidemiologic data suggest that pre-pregnancy maternal obesity may be a risk factor for a variety of birth defects including congenital heart defects. Of the cardiac defects, maternal obesity is specifically associated with an increased risk for both atrial and ventricular septal defects (Cedergren and Kallen, 2003). While the mechanism of this finding is uncertain, the current "epidemic" of obesity in western society makes this association a potentially significant risk factor.

6. Natural history of secundum ASD

There are data indicating that secundum ASD (defined as defects ≥ 4 mm in size) when diagnosed in the first 6 months of life have a tendency to regress in size including the potential for spontaneous closure. In addition, the strongest predictor for spontaneous closure was shown to be *smaller size* at the time of initial diagnosis. In one study, over half of ASD's measuring between 4-5 mm at the time of diagnosis closed spontaneously and an additional 30% regressed to a size considered to be insignificant (≤ 3 mm) (Hanslik et al., 2006). None of the larger defects (> 10 mm) closed spontaneously and over 75% required surgical or device closure (Hanslik et al., 2006). These data certainly suggest that size of the secundum ASD at initial diagnosis directly impacts the natural history and specifically the potential need for closure. Last, the recognition that spontaneous closure of secundum ASD can occur is important, and has obvious implications for prevalence estimates.

7. Future trends regarding secundum ASD prevalence

A key question that remains unanswered is whether the true prevalence of secundum ASD is in fact increasing. Since 1975, the *reported* prevalence of secundum ASD (as well as some of the other common cardiac defects) has increased significantly (Correa et al., 2007; Hoffman & Kaplan, 2002; Wren et al., 2000). Because most of the increase in heart defect prevalence has been seen in asymptomatic infants, (while prevalence in more severe heart defects have been stable), better ascertainment using current color-Doppler echocardiography is clearly felt to be a significant contributing factor. However, there are preliminary evidence that the prevalence of secundum ASD may still be increasing in the most recent time-frame when imaging modalities have *not* changed significantly (Riehle-Colarusso T, unpublished observation). If true, some of the changing demographic factors referred to in this chapter may be contributing factors. However, at the current time, it is not possible to state with certainty whether the actual prevalence of secundum ASD is increasing.

8. Conclusion

This chapter has reviewed data assessing the prevalence of secundum ASD using current imaging modalities and strict guidelines for diagnosis. Secundum ASD is the third most common congenital cardiac defect and, based on the prevalence data reported in this chapter, accounts for greater than 10% of all cardiac defects. In addition, these data show that it is nearly as common as peri-membranous VSD. This chapter has also reviewed the common associations and risk factors that have been identified with secundum ASD. While some of the societal trends mentioned in the review of risk factors for ASD are of interest, knowing whether the prevalence of secundum ASD is in fact, increasing, and if so, what might be causing this, remain speculative at the current time.

9. References

Basson CT, Cowley GS, Solomon SD, et al. (1994). The clinical and genetic spectrum of the Holt-Oram syndrome (heart-hand syndrome). *N Engl J Med* 330:885-889.

Benson DW, Silberbach GM, Kavanaugh-McHugh A, Cottrill C, Zhang Y, et al. (1999). Mutations in the cardiac transcription factor NKX2.5 affect diverse cardiac developmental pathways. *J Clin Invest* 104:1567-1573.

Boldt T, Anderson S, Eronen M. (2002). Outcome of structural heart disease diagnosed in utero. *Scand Cardiovasc J*. 36:73-79.

Botto LD, Lin AE, Riehle-Colarusso T, Malik S, Correa A, and the National Birth Defects Prevention Study. (2007). Seeking Causes: Classifying and Evaluating Congenital Heart Defects in Etiologic Studies. *Birth Defects Research (Part A): Clinical and Molecular Teratology* 79:714-728.

Cedergren MI and Kallen BAJ (2003). Maternal obesity and Infant Heart Defects. *Obesity Research* 11:1065-1071

Correa A, Cragan JD, Kucik ME, et al. (2007). Reporting birth defects surveillance data 1968-2003. *Birth Defects Res A Clin Mol Teratol* 79: 65-186.

Ferencz C, Loffredo CA, Correa-Villasenor A, Wilson PD, eds. (1997). Chapter 10: Atrial Septal Defect: in Genetic & Environmental Risk Factors of Major Cardiovascular Malformations: *The Baltimore-Washington Infant Study 1981-1989*. Futura Publishing Co, Inc. pp 267-283, Armonk, NY.

Ghisla RP, Hannon DW, Meyer RA, et al. (1985). Spontaneous closure of isolate secundum atrial septal defects in infants: an echocardiographic study. *Am Heart J*. 109: I327-I333.

Hanslik A, Pospisil U, Salzer-Muhar U, et al. (2006). Predictors of Spontaneous Closure of Isolated Secundum Atrial Septal Defect in Children: A Longitudinal Study. *Pediatrics* 118: 1560-1565.

Hoffman JI, Kaplan S. (2002). The incidence of congenital heart disease. *J Am Coll Cardiol* 39:1890-1900.

Jacobs JP, Mavroudis C, Jacobs ML, et al. (2004). Lessons learned from the data analysis of the second harvest (1998-2001) of the Society of Thoracic Surgeons (STS) Congenital Heart surgery Database. *Eur J Cardiothorac Surg*. 26: 18-37.

Loffredo C, Wilson P, Ferencz C. (2001). Maternal diabetes: An independent risk factor for major cardiovascular malformations with increased mortality of affected infants. *Teratology* 64:98-106.

Mastroiacovo P, Castilla E, Arpino C, et al. (1999). Congenital malformations in twins: an international study. *Am J Med Genet* 83:117-124.

Mendez HM and Opitz JM (1985). Noonan syndrome: a review. *Am J Med Genet* 21: 493-496.

Mone S, Tillman M, Miller T, et al. (2004). Effects of environmental exposures on the cardiovascular system: prenatal period through adolescence. *Pediatrics* 113: No. 4.

Radzik D, Davignon A, van Doesburg N, et al. (1993). Predictive factors for spontaneous closure of atrial septal defects diagnosed in the first 3 months of life. *J Am Coll Cardiol*. 22:851-853.

Reller MD, Strickland MJ, Riehle-Colarusso T, et al. (2008). Prevalence of Congenital Heart Defects in Metropolitan Atlanta, 1998-2005. *J Pediatr* 153: 807-813.

Riehle-Colarusso T, Strickland MJ, Reller MD, et al. (2007). Improving the quality of surveillance data in congenital heart defects in the metropolitan Atlanta congenital defects program. *Birth Defects Res A Clin Mol Teratol* 79:743-753.

Rosas M, Attie F, Sandoval J, et al. (2004). Atrial septal defect in adults > 40 years old: negative impact of low atrial oxygen saturation. *International Journal of Cardiology* 93:145-155.

Schott JJ, Benson DW, Basson CT, et al. (1998). Congenital Heart Disease caused by mutations in the transcription factor NKX2-5. *Science* 2f81: 108-111.

Wren C, Richmond S, Donaldsdon L. (2000). Temporal variability in birth prevalence of cardiovascular malformations. *Heart* 83:414-419.

Section 3

Creation of ASDs

4

Computer-Aided Automatic Delivery System of High-Intensity Focused Ultrasound for Creation of an Atrial Septal Defect

Hiromasa Yamashita, Gontaro Kitazumi, Keri Kim and Toshio Chiba
National Center for Child Health and Development, Japan

1. Introduction

Several fetal cardiac malformations have been increasingly treated before birth. Fetal cardiac intervention targets an in utero correction of simple intracardiac abnormalities that potentially progress to complex heart diseases in utero, such as fetal critical aortic stenosis that might cause to hypoplastic left heart syndrome (HLHS) and HLHS with restrictive atrial septum leading to irreversible pulmonary vascular damages (Kohl et al., 2000; Marshall et al., 2004; Makikallio et al., 2006). Current operative procedures for correction of fetal restrictive atrial septum with an atrial decompression are still invasive because they, percutaneously and through both the uterine wall and fetal chest walls, require ultrasound-guided maternal puncture into the frequently-pulsating (120-180 counts per minute) cardiac cavity of tiny fetal hearts and to create interatrial communications. Accordingly, these procedures have been reportedly accompanied by serious complications including profound bradycardia, bleeding and hemopericardium, intracardiac thrombus formation, and recurrent in utero closure of the created atrial septal defects.

To establish fetal interatrial communications with minimal adverse effects, we developed an entirely new approach with the use of high intensity focused ultrasound (HIFU) (Fig. 1). HIFU is acoustic modality using ultrasound energy with cavitation and/or coagulation effect focused to operate on an internally targeted tissue without damaging overlying and/or underlying tissues. HIFU has been employed predominantly for non-touch treatment of tumors including prostate cancer, breast cancer and uterine fibroids (Rebillard et al., 2005; Chan et al., 2002; Hengst et al., 2004). Unlike an extensive ablation of stationary tumors, the HIFU ablation to a frequently-pulsating narrow area in the beating and tiny fetal heart requires highly accurate pinpoint delivery in real-time based on computer-aided auto-tracking of atrial septum.

We developed a new automatic delivery system of HIFU with real-time two dimensional-ultrasound (2D-US) imaging analysis. Features of this system are 1) automatic detection of heartbeat rates, 2) automatic estimation of atrial septum position, 3) automatic generation of HIFU delivery timing and we did feasibility study for creation of an atrial septal defect using the beating heart of anesthetized adult rabbits.

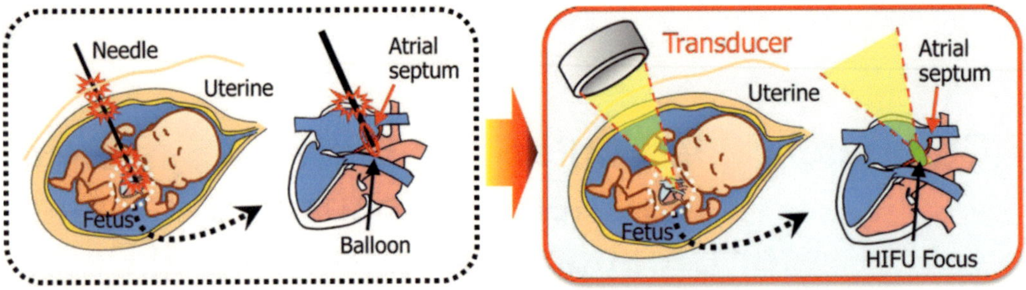

Fig. 1. New approach with HIFU to correct cardiac morphologic abnormalities less invasively.

2. Methods

2.1 System configuration

The system configuration of the computer-aided automatic delivery system of HIFU consists of predominantly 5 parts (Fig. 2). The first one is a HIFU delivery device which comprises a monocoque spherical shaped piezo transducer and a diagnostic 2D-US imaging probe mounted on the transducer. The tomographic images are taken by the probe including the focal point of the transducer. The curvature radius of the transducer is 40 mm, and the focal point is located 40-mm apart from the edge face of the transducer. The focal point is an elliptical in shape (0.6-mm wide, 5.0-mm long). The second part is a diagnostic 2D-US imaging equipment (En-Visor C HD, Philips, Andover. MA) to scan a cardiac four-chamber view by 2D-US imaging probe (s12, Philips, Andover. MA). The equipment outputs gray

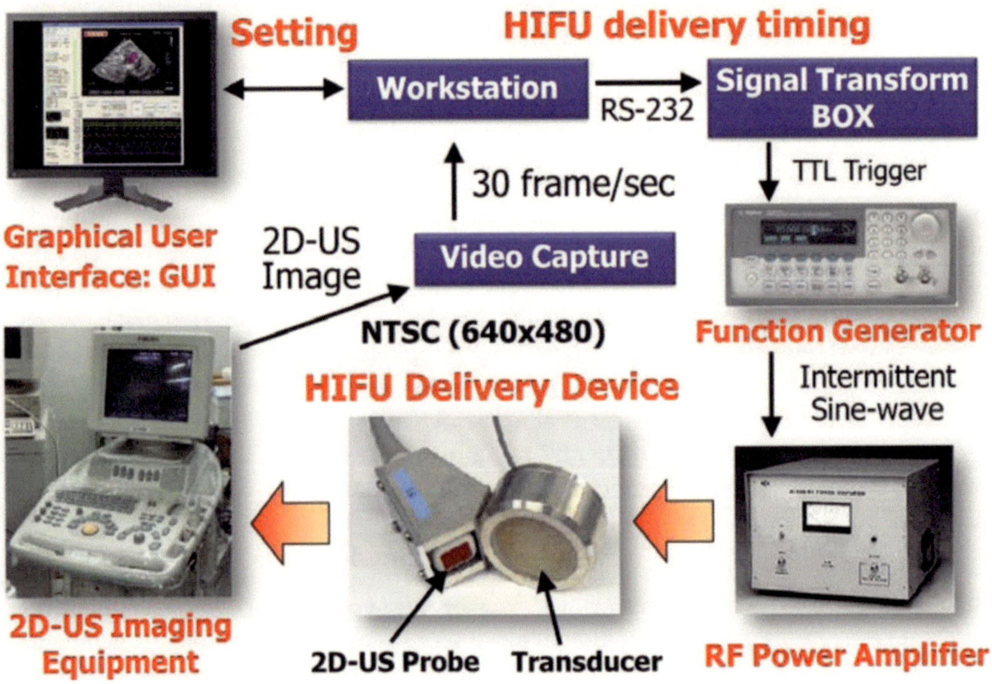

Fig. 2. System configuration of the computer-aided automatic HIFU energy delivery.

scale NTSC-video data (640x480 pixels) into the workstation with 30 frames/sec through a video capture (ADVC-55, Canopus, Kobe) and IEEE1394 cable. The third part is a workstation (HP xw8400, Windows XP x64, Intel Xeon 2.33 GHz, Quad Core, 16GB RAM, DirectX9.0c) to analyze an input 2D-US tomographic image of cardiac four-chamber with our original real-time HIFU delivery control algorithm. The workstation detects heartbeat rates, estimates atrial septum positions, and generates HIFU delivery timing by RS-232 interface into a signal transform box automatically. The fourth part is a function generator (Agilent 33220A, Agilent technologies, Santa Clara, CA) to output intermittent sine-wave with certain frequency and voltage into the fifth part, and RF power amplifier (AG1012, T&C power Conversion Inc., Rochester, NY). The timing to drive the transducer by amplified sine-wave is determined by TTL trigger from the signal transform box. Automatic HIFU delivery is accomplished by some adjusting with various parameters. This setting is done through a graphical user interface on the monitor by surgeons (Fig. 3).

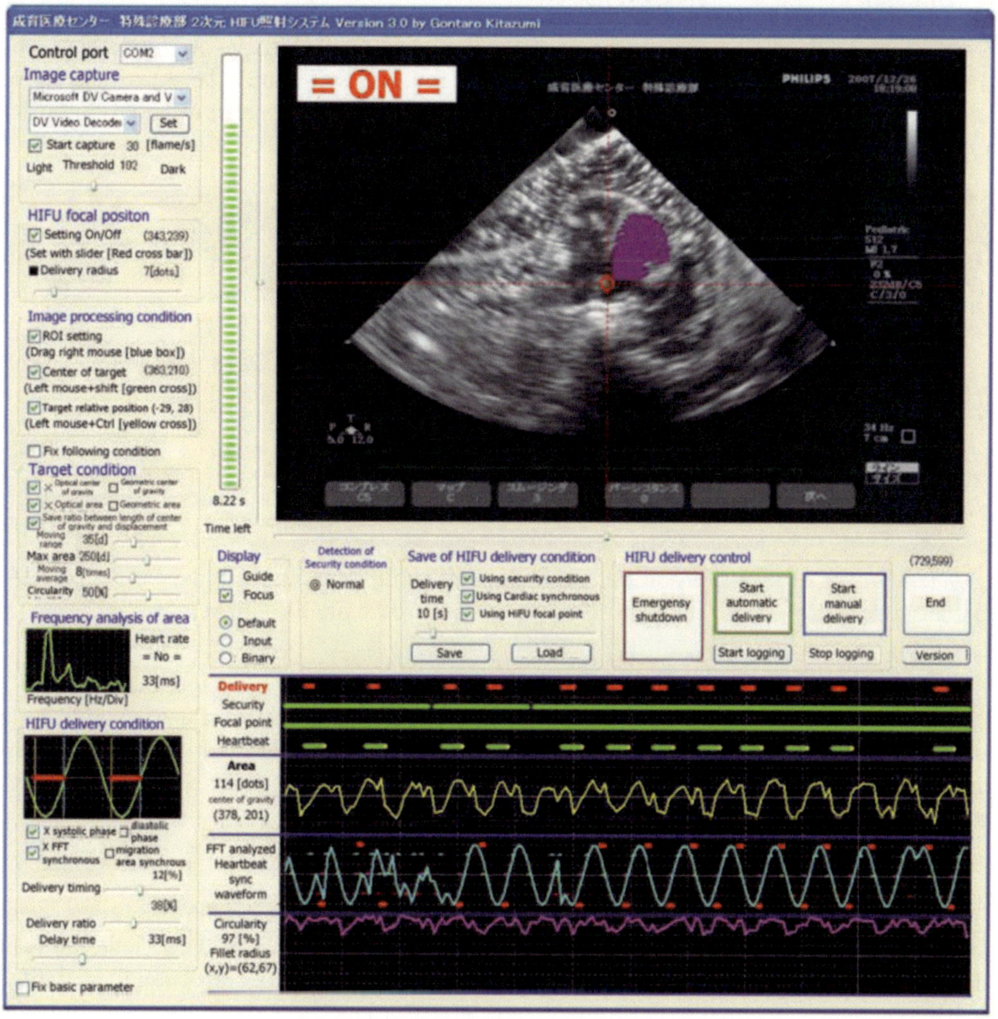

Fig. 3. Graphical user interface for setting, adjusting and monitoring of automatic HIFU delivery.

2.2 Automatic detection of heartbeat rates

The atrial septum, which is a target of this system to be perforated, repeats expansion, shrinkage and movement with heartbeat. It is assumed that the best timing to perforate an atrial septum safely by HIFU delivery system is when the atrial septum is expanded most. However, because the atrial septum has less features in 2D-US image, it is difficult to detect its movement directly. Therefore, using the fact that atrial septum expands when ventricle contracts, we tried to detect the timing when the left ventricle contracts most, which is easy to detect by 2D-US image. The left ventricular movement of expansion and shrinkage are caused by heartbeats, and its variation can be associated with the change of the left ventricular area in 2D-US image. In this paper, we utilized the automatic detection of the heartbeat period by the following procedures.

1. Setting of Region of Interest (ROI)

We set a rectangular ROI surrounding the left ventricle of 2D-US image on the display while confirming four chamber view of 2D-US image (Fig. 4(A)). ROI should be set so that the left ventricle, which repeats expansion, shrinkage and movement, doesn't protrude it, and ROI should be the smallest to minimize calculation cost in the image processing.

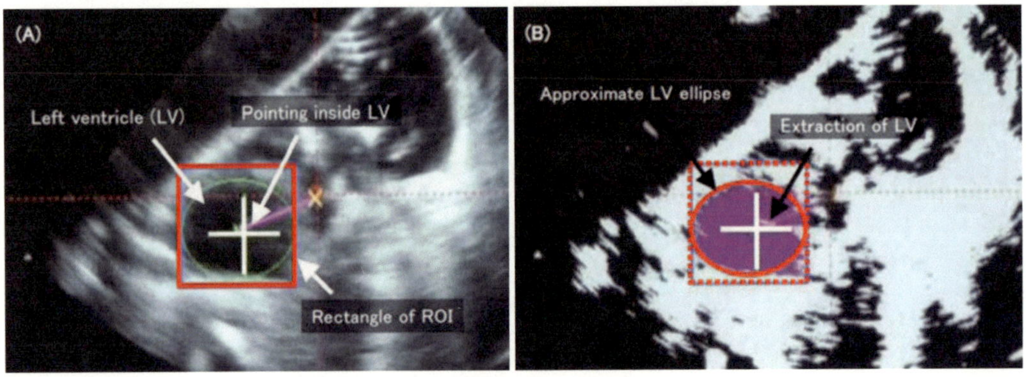

Fig. 4. (A) Setting of ROI and point of inside the left ventricle (LV). (B) Binary image of 2D-US image, extraction of the left ventricle area and approximate LV ellipse.

2. Pointing of inside the left ventricle

Using 2D-US binarized image by white and black pixels, and the central of inside the left ventricle is pointed by manual in ROI to set target region of the left ventricle to be tracked (Fig. 4(A)). The amount of black pixels which is communicating with the point in ROI is extracted automatically as a left ventricular area.

3. Adjustment of a threshold value in binarization of 2D-US image

2D-US image for the image processing is expressed in gray scale of 256 brightness levels. The threshold value for binarization should be adjusted between 0 and 255 levels so as to extract the left ventricular area adequately. When it is adjusted most adequately, a shape of the left ventricle is approximated an ellipse (Fig. 4(B)). However depending on threshold, the outside of the left ventricle is detected by error and, to the contrary, inside of the left ventricle is not detected. These errors influence precision of the left ventricular area and calculation of its geometry described below. Overestimation or underestimation of the left ventricular area causes "undetectable". In our system the threshold value is adjusted empirically considering actual 2D-US image so that a ratio to be "undetectable" becomes as small as possible.

4. Frequency analysis of the left ventricular area variation

It becomes possible to take samples about variation of the left ventricular area at frequency of 30 times per seconds when the area is extracted adequately. This is because the variation of areas includes heartbeats, low-frequency component by breathing and high-frequency component by noise when 2D-US image is acquired and transferred to the workstation. It is necessary to remove these components by filtering with a small calculation cost. Our system uses the moving average calculation with 8 past samples to remove the low frequency component and the simplicity mean calculation with 2 past samples to remove the high-frequency component. Using fast Fourier transformation the system calculates heartbeat period, frequency and period from 64 past samples without some noises automatically.

2.3 Automatic estimation of atrial septum

As mentioned previously, the atrial septum has less features in 2D-US image which is difficult to detect its position by image processing directly. Therefore the system is set to delivery HIFU only, when position of the atrial septum can be estimated from position and shape of the left ventricle, which is easy to be detected in 2D-US image, and its position corresponds to the focal point of HIFU delivery by a fixed transducer. In this study an automatic estimation of the atrial septum is realized according to following procedures. In addition, the positional information of estimated atrial septum is used as a safety conditional for HIFU delivery based on the allowable error.

1. Position adjustment of HIFU transducer

The transducer and 2D-US probe are fixed physically for one HIFU delivery device. At first, the focal point of HIFU delivery is confirmed precisely by 2D-US image when HIFU is delivering to a low decrement polymer-coated rubber with the acoustic impedance (Acoustic standoff, Eastek Corporation, Tokyo, Japan) that is approximately equivalent to a human body (Fig. 5). The resolution of this 2D-US image around the focus is about 0.5 mm in the direction that throws the beam and about 0.2 mm in the depth direction. We mark a circle to the focal position on this 2D-US image supported by orthogonally-crossed guide lines (Fig. 6(A)). The position and the posture of HIFU delivery device is fixed by manual so that position of the atrial septum corresponds to the focal point of HIFU transducer in the timing when left ventricle shrinks most.

2. Making template information

As well as preceding clause, we mark a cross on the atrial septum of the timing when the left ventricle shrinks most by manual operation and define the coordinate with (XAt, YAt). In addition, we define the fillet diameter of the left ventricle shape approximated by a ellipse with (RXt, RYt) and the coordinate of center of gravity position with (XGt, YGt), and use these parameters for the image analysis in the next clause as template information to estimate the atrial septum position (Fig. 6(B)).

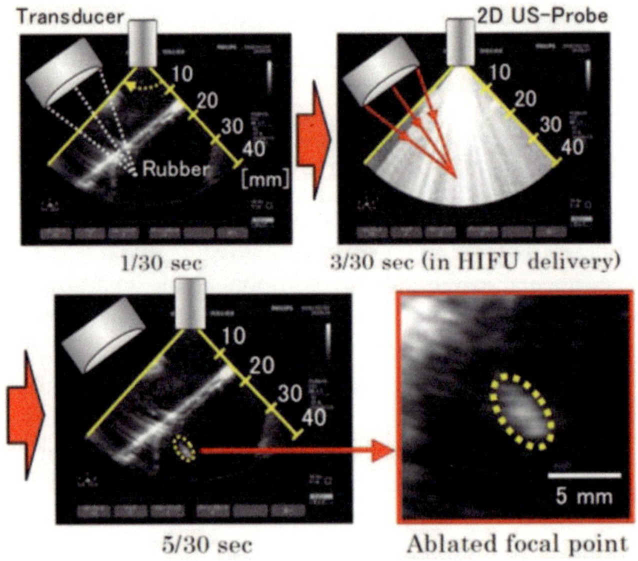

Fig. 5. Confirmation of ablated focal point by HIFU delivery on 2D-US image. Ablated focal point is ellipsoid of 5-mm long and 2-mm wide.

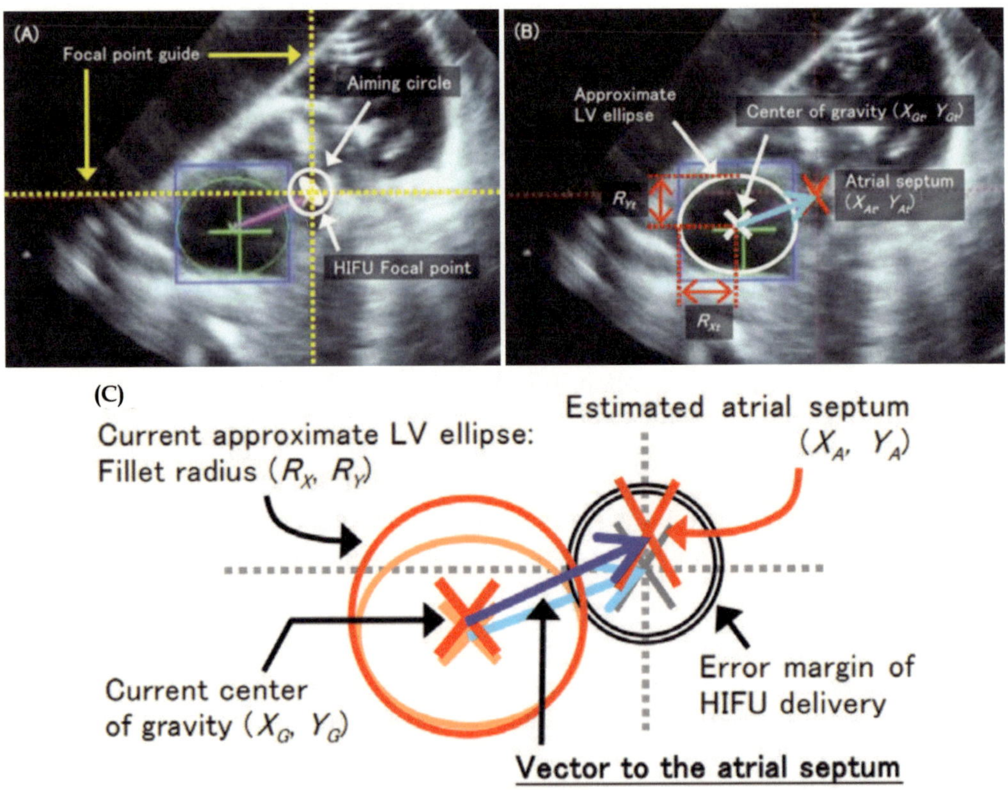

Fig. 6. (A) Pointing focus of HIFU with X-Y guide lines on the 2D-US image. (B) Determination of template parameters by pointing of atrial septum and getting fillet radius

of approximate LV ellipse (RXt, RYt) and its center of gravity (XGt, YGt) when the left ventricle is minimum. (C) Automatic estimation of atrial septum position (XA, YA) with geometric ratio between current information (fillet radius and center of gravity position) and template parameters. If estimated position is in the error margin circle of HIFU focus, HIFU delivery is allowed.

3. Geometric estimation of the atrial septum position

Using the left ventricular fillet diameter (RX, RY) and the geometric center of gravity position (XG, YG) detected in 30 frames per seconds, template fillet diameter (RXt, RYt) and template geometric center of gravity position (XGt, YGt). We estimate current atrial septum position (XA, YA) by formula (1) automatically (Fig. 6(C)). HIFU delivery is permitted only when the position (XA, YA) is in a circle around (XAt, YAt) for allowable error.

$$\begin{cases} XA = XG + (XAt + XGt) \times RX / RXt \\ YA = YG + (YAt + YGt) \times RY / RYt \end{cases} \quad (1)$$

2.4 Definition of HIFU delivery timing

It is determined the timing when HIFU should be delivered by analysis of the four chamber view in 2D-US image. However, there is the delay time (TD) constantly between acquisition of 2D-US image, image transformation by the video capture, image analysis with the workstation, trigger output to a function generator, sinusoidal amplification in the RF power amplifier and HIFU delivery by a transducer. It is about 33 ms in this system, which is just equal to the delay for 1 frame of 2D-US image. Therefore based on the image analysis results HIFU delivery is enabled the timing when the left ventricle shrinks most by the trigger of HIFU delivery at the time of "TS-TD", which deducted the delay time from the predicted time that left ventricle shrinks most (TS) (Fig. 7).

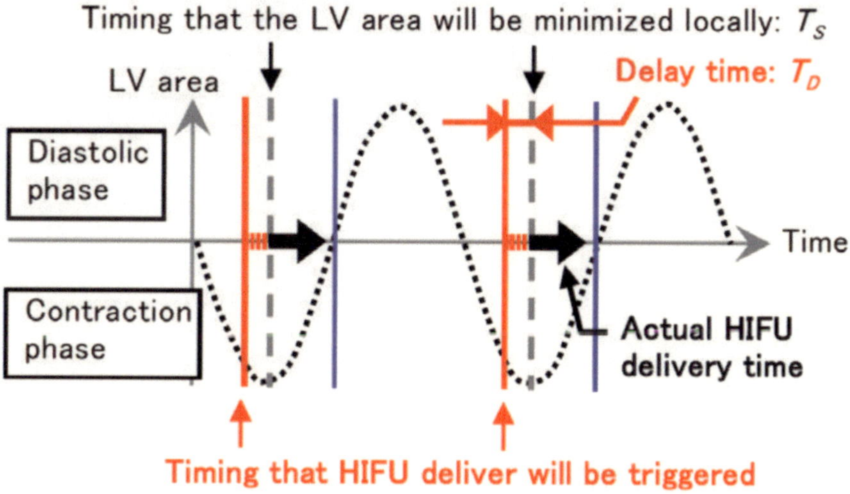

Fig. 7. Definition of HIFU delivery starting trigger timing with total delay time in the system. The timing is the delay time TD before the timing TS that the left ventricle area will be minimized locally.

2.5 Security condition for HIFU delivery

HIFU delivery is conducted based on the timing when the left ventricle shrinks most in consideration of the delay time in the system. In order to avoid some issues, caused by various factors and disturbances, to deliver HIFU outside of the allowable circle The system is permitted to delivery HIFU as far as meeting following security conditions so as to avoid "shooting by mistake", which means that HIFU delivery is outside the allowable limit of error radius and ablated point is overshot the actual atrial septum, even if the point is inside the allowable limit of error radius (Fig. 8).

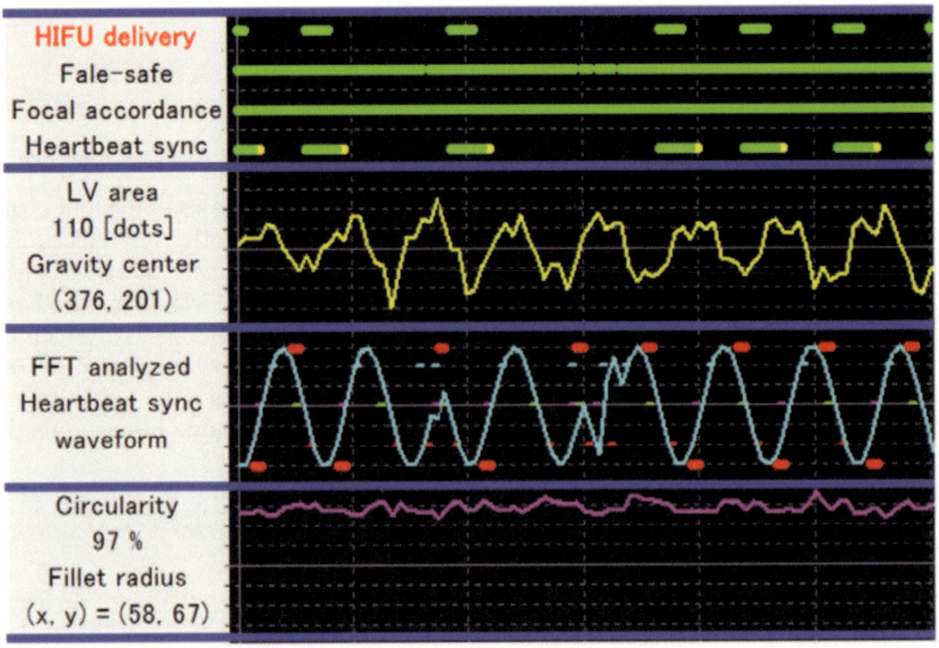

Fig. 8. Monitoring of HIFU delivery condition defined by focal accordance, area of LV, heartbeat synchronous and circularity of LV.

1. The upper limit of movement distance of the left ventricular geometric center of gravity
2. The maximum value of the left ventricle area
3. Success or failure of the heartbeat cycle detection by fast Fourier transformation
4. The minimum value of the ellipsoid roundness, which is approximate shape of the left ventricle
5. Whether an estimated position of the atrial septum is inside focal allowance limits of error or not

These conditional thresholds are settable individually, and we can select any conditions. Delivery frequency decreases if the conditions are strict. On the other hand, it increases if the conditions are easy. However, we have only a rough index for optimal parameters because individual difference is large by the delivered target of HIFU. Therefore, it is necessary to judge during securing safety as the trigger off for HIFU delivery while watching the temporal change in HIFU delivery condition on the display whether you can irradiate it more effectively, the parameters are appropriate, or more effective delivery is possible.

3. *In vivo* experiment

3.1 Purpose

In this experiment, we confirmed feasibility of our computer-aided automatic delivery system of HIFU to perform atrial septal defect creation of animals in vivo. We used four healthy animals (Japanese white rabbit, male, 2.8 kg) with cardiac pulsation under anesthesia. Their bodies are slightly larger than our practical target fetus.

3.2 Methods

We tested HIFU delivery to adult rabbits of which limbs were fixed to the operating table. This is because it was covered by flat breast bone, and HIFU reflected the heart of the rabbit. We tried HIFU delivery in a state exposed with rabbit's heart by a median section and under the environment that which heart moves during the pulmonary respiration by the respirator unlike intrauterine fetuses. In the case of practical intrauterine fetuses, their undeveloped breast bone does not damp HIFU and they don't breathe with lung. We performed this experiment in the following procedures strictly in accordance with the rule that the animal executive committee in National Center for Child Health and Development.

1. Four adult rabbits (Japanese White, 2.8 kg, male) were anesthetized with xylazine (5 mg/kg IM) and isoflurane by inhalation.
2. After endotracheal intubation or tracheostomy placement, anesthesia was maintained on the mechanical ventilation with isoflurane and oxygen inhalation (20 cycles/min, 240 ml/cycle).
3. ECG, arterial blood pressure/oxygen saturation, and end-tidal carbon dioxide concentration were monitored intraoperatively in real time.
4. The animals underwent median sternotomy to expose the heart, chest cavities were filled with buffering gel on both sides. The heart beats was set in the direct contact with a silicone sheet-bottomed tank filled with degassed water (37°C) (Fig. 9).
5. A HIFU transducer combined with a diagnostic 2D-US imaging probe was fixed on a two-directional (X-Y) linear stage with a pivot hinge placed on the tank which was manually steered, so that the HIFU focal point could be roughly located on the atrial septum of the beating heart.
6. Various parameters for HIFU delivery were specified.
7. Automatic HIFU delivery was carried out with this system.
8. After HIFU delivery, we confirm whether new blood flows is generated across the atrial septum using color Doppler echocardiography by the diagnostic 2D-US imaging equipment.

9. After this experiment, we inject pentobarbital into a peripheral venous path and sacrifice the rabbits.

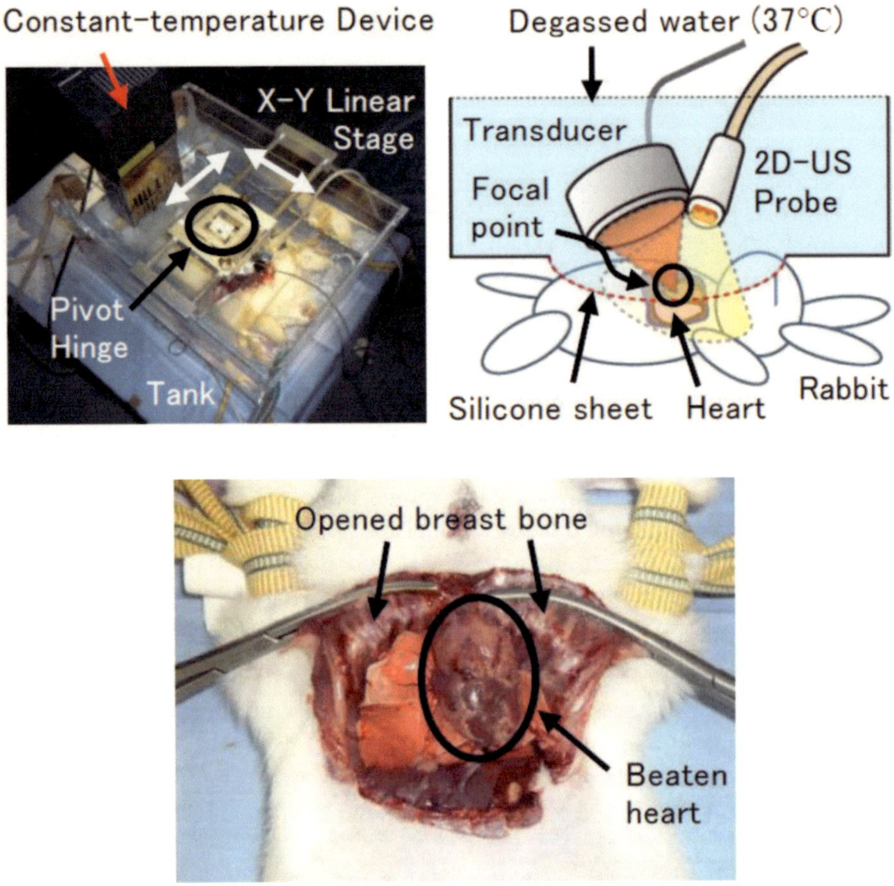

Fig. 9. Experimental setup using an adult rabbit. HIFU delivery was done through a silicone sheet at the bottom of the degassed water tank.

3.3 HIFU delivery condition

The waveform output from a function generator is observable with an oscilloscope, which is amplified by RF power amplifier and is input to a transducer. In this experiment, the input waveform was sine wave of 3.3 MHz, 160 Vpp and 6.5 kW/cm^2.

For the total HIFU delivery time in one trial, we set three seconds from experiences of the prior pilot study. The allowable limit of error radius of HIFU delivery spot is set to the same value in all trial so that it was with the smallest circle which a focus shape of HIFU was fit into on a display.

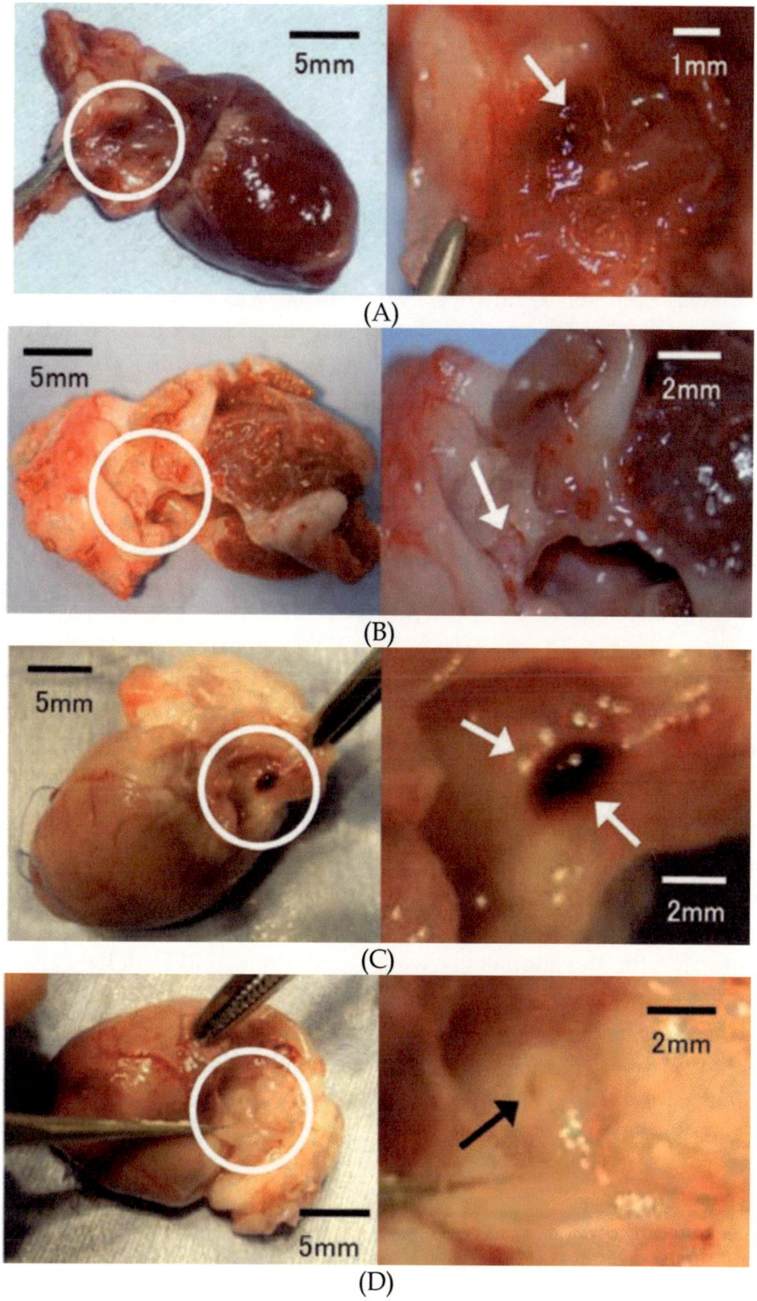

Fig. 10. Heart specimens ablated with HIFU delivery. Left images are gross appearances of the inadvertent ablation with opening. Right images are magnifications of the area ablated by HIFU deliveries. (A) A small opening was made in the posterior wall of the left atrium. (B) Atrial septum apparently remained non-penetrated with mere coagulation changes. (C) Non-penetrated small hole was made on the atrial septum with hematoma formation. (D) Non-penetrated small hole was made on the atrial septum accurately.

The HIFU delivery began at the moment when a surgeon pushed the button for beginning of automatic delivery on a display and came back to the standby state when 3-seconds HIFU delivery was completed in total.

3.4 Results

Four rabbits were euthanized after HIFU delivery, and dissected their isolated hearts and observed around the atrial septum (Fig. 10(A) - (D)). In the first trial, it took 23 seconds from beginning of automatic HIFU delivery to the end (Fig. 10(A)). The penetration of the tissue in the chamber was completed, however the position was missed from the atrial septum toward posterior parietal side, which is the left atrium side. In the second trial, it took 57 seconds by the end (Fig. 10(B)). A cauterization spot was found on the atrial septum in pinpoint, however the HIFU delivery did not achieve a penetration. In the third trial, it took 44 seconds by the end (Fig. 10(C)). The perforation on the atrial septum was confirmed, however it did not achieved a penetration. In addition a hematoma-like change was found beside a perforation spot. In the last trial, it took 46 seconds by the end (Fig. 10(D)). The perforation on the atrial septum was confirmed, however it did not achieve a penetration. Unlike the third trial the hematoma was not found.

4. Discussion

In this study, we developed automatic delivery system of HIFU based on real-time 2D-US imaging analysis. In in vivo experiment we confirmed pinpoint delivery of HIFU to the pulsating atrial septum within beating hearts of anesthetized adult rabbits.

In the field of cardiology, HIFU was investigated as a promising device to treat arrhythmia, relieve valvular stenosis and ameliorate obstructive hypertrophic cardiomyopathy. HIFU also enables us to create defects in cardiac tissues such as ventricles or cusp of the aortic valve in vitro or ex vivo (Otsuka et al., 2005; Fujikura et al., 2006; Lee et al., 2000; Xu et al., 2004; Strickberger et al., 1999). Particularly in fetal cardiac intervention, less invasiveness of HIFU is effective for the mother as well. In addition, HIFU delivery can be a actual operative method with security, a short time and low cost. Our new system is useful for an approach into the heart chamber with more safety owing to detection of a heartbeat cycle only from 2D-US four chamber view without other measurement instruments and estimation of atrial septum position pulsating with heartbeats and breathing for more effective HIFU delivery.

4.1 Detection of heartbeat

In order to obtain heartbeat information, it is common to use an electrocardiogram (ECG). There is a reported study to try the treatment of arrhythmias using the HIFU delivery triggered by ECG (Strickberger et al., 1999). However, it is difficult to isolate only ECG of fetus from a maternal ECG definitely although fetal ECG monitoring is technically quite demanding because ECG of fetus is obtained only through the mother. Therefore, the method to detect the heartbeat cycle of fetus only from real-time 2D-US image in our system is thought to be appropriate for clinical application from convenient point of view. However, based on the image processing, the amount of calculation is larger and delay time is longer than ECG signal analysis. This is because arrhythmic development is expected, and heartbeat cycle collapses with a diseased heart. It is better that the delay time is short to detect arrhythmic development quickly. We had a plan to introduce the system with fetal ECG together in near future.

4.2 Estimation of atrial septum

About the estimation of the atrial septum position, although the surgeon confirmed it by monitoring before HIFU delivery in vivo experimental qualitatively, ablated point was not so overshot the atrial septum, of which position was estimated from 2D-US image. However, when the 2D-US image was not clear, the left ventricular position and shape were not obtained precisely. There were some cases that estimation of the atrial septum was impossible. Consequently, HIFU delivery was not permitted by security conditions in this case. We were able to avoid shooting by mistake outside the allowable limit of error radius in 2D-US image. Also, we calculated geometric ratio between the left ventricular center of gravity position and the approximate fillet diameter for "correct answer" which a surgeon sets by manual operation as template information, however the procedure is limited on 2D plane. We don't consider that the heartbeat includes movement and transformation (expansion, shrinkage and distortion) not only in 2D plane (X-Y plane), but also in the depth direction (Z-axis direction). It depends on how detection of the heartbeat and the estimation of the atrial septum position are accurate what appropriate four chamber view is acquired. The detection of the heartbeat from the extraction of the left ventricular area on 2D-US image is no more than approximation. Even if the focal point is inside allowable limit of error radius in 2D-US image, the HIFU delivery results in shooting by mistake three-dimensionally because prior confirmation of the HIFU focal size and shape, fixation of the HIFU delivery device, and setting of the parameters about HIFU delivery condition were performed on the basis of 2D-US image only. This is the major reason of the HIFU delivery position error. For the solution of this issue, at least when HIFU delivery device is fixed on target we should use a three-dimensional ultrasound (3D-US) probe to recognize detail of 3D positional relationship between the focal point and the actual atrial septum in beating heart for more accurate focal position alignment. It is expected that performance of the 3D-US diagnostic equipment improves to acquire and analyze 3D-US voxel data in real time directly, which leads drastically higher precision of HIFU delivery with our system in near future.

In addition, the real intrauterine fetus is floating in the amniotic fluid and is movable three-dimensionally. During surgery, the fetus doesn't exercise spontaneously because both mother and fetus are under anesthesia, however we have to track not only movement of the atrial septum but also the fetal movement of oneself. That is to say in addition to 2D-US for four chamber view of the heart. We need 3D-US to track movement of intrauterine fetus three-dimensionally. At the same time it is important to move HIFU delivery device itself mechanically to track fetal wide movement in utero (Koizumi et al., 2008).

4.3 In vivo experiment

We tried HIFU delivery to the animals which imitated intrauterine fetuses, however the results didn't achieved both delivery efficiency and delivery accuracy of HIFU. The only one trial perforated tissue in the beating chamber, and the perforated point was on the adjacent tissue of the atrial septum. On the other hand, the three trials ablated just the atrial septum, and no perforations were generated. The HIFU delivery efficiency depends on the ratio of delivery time in one heartbeat and the total time to complete preset HIFU delivery in each trial. In all trials, we set the same delivery conditions on a respirator, size (weight) of the animal, the allowable limit of error radius around HIFU focal point, and the total HIFU delivery time. However, there were individual differences in animals' heartbeat cycle and 2D-US image of the left ventricle, and also, we found small differences in relative position relationship between animal body and HIFU delivery device because we made adjustments to delivery setting in each trial. Therefore, the variation occurred in the total time to complete preset HIFU delivery in each trial. To increase the safety, the shorter delivery ratio in one heartbeat and more strict security conditions are required. However, if the total time lead to longer to complete preset HIFU delivery, the one HIFU delivery interval gets longer, which results in no perforation of the tissue due to diffusion of converged HIFU energy into intracardiac blood flow. HIFU delivery frequency around 3.3 MHz may cause heating effect and/or mechanical (cavitation) effect. If the perforation of tissue is caused by only mechanical effect of cavitation, we need not consider the diffusion of the HIFU energy in to the blood flow. In order to avoid cooling effect by the blood flow, it is more useful to take advantege of mechanical effect of cavitation positively. However, it is necessary to progress clarification about which is dominant heating effect or mechanical effect of cavitation by detailed simulation and local observation around the focal point. When heating effect is dominant, we should lengthen the delivery ratio in one heartbeat to raise HIFU delivery efficiency and make continuous HIFU delivery by loose of security conditions. However, the security of HIFU delivery tuens down by contraries and the possibility is reduced to be delivered in the point that we aim at. Assurance of security is in a relation of the trade-off with HIFU delivery efficiency, and balancing both is not easy. For safe and secure HIFU delivery we will progress further validation to investigate optimal HIFU delivery conditions from both hardware and software point of view.

5. Conclusion

We developed computer-aided automatic delivery system of HIFU for creation of an atrial septal defect which perforates tissue in the intracardiac chamber for less invasive cardiac intervention of intrauterine fetuses. In vivo experiment using animals, by only 2D-US image of four chamber view, it was possible to detect heartbeat period, estimate the atrial septum position, and determine HIFU delivery timing in real-time under heartbeats.

In near future, we will aim at the clinical application as a minimal invasive surgical system in order to improve precision improvement of the focus positioning of HIFU delivery and improvement of HIFU energy efficiency to intracardiac tissue.

6. Acknowledgement

We wish to thank Akiko Suzuki for help in preparing the manuscript. And a part of this work was supported by Grant Program for Child Health and Development (16-3) administrated by Ministry of Health, Labour and Welfare of Japan.

7. References

Chan, AH., Fujimoto, VY., Moore, DE., Martin, RW. & Vaezy, S.(2002). An image-guided high intensity focused ul-trasound device for uterine fibroids treatment, Medical Physics, Vol. 29, Issue 11, pp. 2611-2611

Fujikura, K., Otsuka, R., Kalisz, A., Ketterling, JA., Jin, Z., Sciacca, RR., Marboe, CC.,Wang, J., Muratore, R., Feleppa, EJ. & Homma, S.(2006). Effects of ultrasonic exposure parameters on myocardial lesions induced by high-intensity focused ultrasound, Journal of Ultrasound in Medecine, Vol. 25, No. 11, pp. 1375-1386

Hengst, SA., Ehrenstein, T., Herzog, H., Beck, A., Utz-Billing, I., David, M., Felix, R., Ricke, J.(2004), Magnetic resonance tomography guided focused ultrasound surgery (MRgFUS) in tumor therapy--a new noninvasive therapy option, Radiology, Vol. 44, Issue 4, pp. 339-346

Kohl, T., Sharland, G., Alllan, LD., Gembruch,U., Chaoui, R., Lopes, LM., Zielinsky, P., Huhta, J. & Silverman, NH.(2000). World experience of percutaneous ultrasound-guided balloon valvuloplasty in human fetuses with severe aortic valve obstruction, American Journal of Cardiology, Vol. 85, pp. 1230-1233

Koizumi, N., Ota, K., Lee, D., Yoshizawa, S., Ito, A., Kaneko, Y., Yoshinaka, K., Matsumoto, Y., & Mitsuishi, M.(2008). Feed-forward controller for the integrated non-invasive ultrasound diagnosis and treatment. Journal of Robotics and Mechatronics, Vol. 20, No. 1, pp. 89-97

Lee, LA., Simon, C., Bove, LE., Mosca, RS., Ebbini, ES., Abrams, GD. & Ludomirsky, A.(2000). High intensity focused ultrasound effect on cardiac tissues: Potential for Clinical application. Echocardiography, Vol. 17, Issue 6, pp. 563-566

Makikallio, K., McElhinney, DB., Levine, JC., Marx, GR., Colan, SD., Marshall, AC., Lock JE., Marcus, EN. & Tworetzky, W.(2006). Fetal Aortic valve stenosis and the evolution of hypoplastic left heart syndrome patient selection for fetal intervention, Circulation, Vol. 113, pp. 1401-1405

Marshall, AC., van der Velde, ME., Tworetzky,W., Gomez, CA., Wilkins-Haung, L., Benson,CB., Jennings, RW. & Lock, JE.(2004). Creation of an atrial septal defect in utero for fetuses with hypoplastic left heart syndrome and intact or highly restrictive atrial septum, Circulation, Vol. 110, pp. 253-258

Otsuka, R., Fujikura, K., Hirata, K., Pulerwitz, T., Oe, Y., Suzuki, T., Sciacca, R., Marboe, C., Wang, J., Burkhoff, D., Muratore, R., Lizzi, FL. & Homma, S.(2005). In vitro ablation of cardiac valves using high-intensity focused ultrasound, Ultrasound in Medicine & Biology, Vol. 31, Issue 1, pp. 109-114

Rebillard, X., Gelet, A., Davin, JL., Soulie, M., Prapotnich, D., Cathelineau, X., Rozet, F. & Vallancien, G.(2005). Transrectal high-intensity focused ultrasound in the treatment of localized prostate cancer, Journal of Endourology, Vol. 2005, Issue 6, pp. 693-701

Strickberger, SA., Tokano, T., Kluiwstra, JUA., Morady, F. & Cain, C.(1999). Extracardiac ablation of the canine atrioventricular junction by use of high-intensity focused ultrasound,Circulation, Vol. 100, pp. 203-208

Xu, Z., Ludmirsky, A., Eun, LY., Hall, TL., Tran, BC., Fowlkes, JB. & Cain, CA.(2004). Controlled ultrasound tissue erosion, IEEE transactions on ultrasonics, ferroelectrics, and frequency control, Vol. 51, Issue 6, pp. 726–736

Yamashita, H., Ishii, T., Ishiyama, A., Nakayama, N., Miyoshi, T., Miyamoto, Y., Kitazumi, G., Katsuike, Y., Okazaki, M., Azuma, T., Fujisaki, M., Takamoto, S. & Chiba, T.(2008). Computer-aided Delivery of High-Intensity Focused Ultrasound (HIFU) for Creation of an Atrial Septal Defect In vivo, Lecture Notes in Computer Science(LNCS), Vol. 5128, pp. 300–310

Section 4

Transcatheter Closure of ASD

5

Historical Aspects of Transcatheter Occlusion of Atrial Septal Defects

Srilatha Alapati and P. Syamasundar Rao
University of Texas at Houston Medical School, Houston, TX, USA

1. Introduction

Following the description of surgical closure of atrial septal defect (ASD) in early 1950s (Bigelow et al., 1950; Lewis et al., 1953; Gibbon, 1953), it rapidly became a standard therapy of ASDs. Surgical closure of ostium secundum ASDs is safe and effective with negligible mortality (Murphy et al., 1990; Galal et al., 1994; Pastorek et al., 1994), but the morbidity associated with sternotomy/thoracotomy, cardiopulmonary bypass and potential for postoperative complications cannot be avoided. Other disadvantages of surgical therapy are the expense associated with surgical correction, residual surgical scar and psychological trauma to the patients and/or the parents. Presumably because of these reasons, several groups of cardiologists embarked upon developing transcatheter methods of closure of the ASD. The studies of King (King & Mills, 1974; Mills & King, 1976; King et al., 1976), Rashkind (Rashkind, 1975; Rashkind & Cuaso, 1977; Rashkind, 1983) and their associates paved the way for the future development of transcatheter ASD device occlusion methodology. In this chapter, history of development of ASD closure devices will be reviewed. Historical development for occlusion of patent foramen ovale (PFO) will be briefed at the end of the chapter.

2. Closure of atrial septal defects

Historical aspects of closure of atrial septal defect will be reviewed in this section.

2.1 King and Mill's device

King and his associates were successful in occluding the ASD via a transcatheter delivered occluding device and were the first in doing so and reported their studies in mid 70s (King & Mills, 1974; Mills & King, 1976; King et al., 1976). This device is composed of paired, Dacron-covered stainless steel umbrellas (Figure 1A) collapsed into a capsule at the tip of a catheter. A number of sizes of the umbrella were manufactured. King & Mills (1974) initially attempted this technique in experimental animal models. ASDs were created by a punch biopsy technique in adult dogs. Successful device deployment was achieved in five of nine dogs in whom the procedure was attempted. Complete closure of the ASD and endothelialization of the implanted umbrellas was observed during the follow-up.

Following this experience in the dog model, the technique was extended to human subjects (Mills & King, 1976; King et al., 1976). Stretched ASD diameter was measured by balloon sizing (King et al., 1978) and a device 10 mm larger than the stretched ASD diameter is selected for deployment. The device delivery catheter is inserted through the saphenous vein at the sapheno-femoral venous junction by cut-down. The catheter tip is positioned into the left atrium through the ASD. The distal umbrella is extruded in the body of the left atrium and the catheter withdrawn into the right atrium. Then, the distal (left atrial) umbrella is fixed against the left side of the atrial septum and the proximal (right atrial) umbrella is opened in the right atrium. The umbrellas are locked to each other with a special locking mechanism. After the device is in place, the obturator wire is unscrewed and withdrawn, thus releasing the device.

Eighteen patients were taken to the catheterization laboratory and ten (56%) of these were considered suitable candidates for device closure. Successful implantation of the device was accomplished in five (50%) patients. Their ages were 17 to 75 years with a median of 24. The stretched ASD diameter was 18 to 26 mm by balloon sizing. Ostium secundum ASD with left-to-right shunt was present in four patients. The fifth patient had an atrial defect with presumed paradoxical embolism and a stroke. Symptoms improved and the heart size decreased during observed follow-up. Repeat cardiac catheterization data did not show shunts by oximetry. However, trivial shunts were observed by hydrogen curves. In a 27 year follow up study, 4 patients remain alive with closed defects and there had been no adverse events related to the device. The deceased patient died from Hodgkin's disease and a cerebral vascular accident 9 years after device closure (King & Mills, 2010).

Although these results were encouraging, King and his associates did not continue their use nor did any other investigator, to our knowledge, pursued the technique. It may be presumed that this may be related to the need for a large delivery sheath and complicated maneuvering required for implantation of the device.

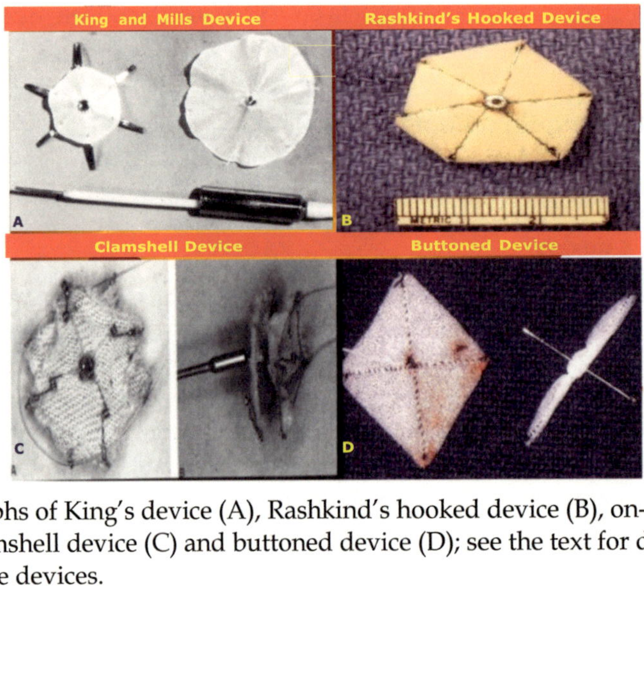

Fig. 1. Photographs of King's device (A), Rashkind's hooked device (B), on-face and side views of the clamshell device (C) and buttoned device (D); see the text for detailed description of the devices.

2.2 Rashkind's devices

Rashkind developed a slightly different type of ASD closure device. Rashkind's investigations appear to be parallel to those of King and Mills (Rashkind et al., 1985). The first Rashkind umbrella consisted of three stainless-steel arms covered with medical grade foam (Rashkind & Cuaso, 1977). The central ends of the stainless-steel arms are attached to miniature springs, which in turn are welded to a small central hub. The outer end of the stainless steel arm ended in a miniature "fish" hook. Rashkind subsequently modified this umbrella such that there are six stainless steel arms with the alternate arms carrying the hook (Figure 1B). He also designed an elaborate centering mechanism, which consisted of five arms bent to produce a gentle outward curve. The umbrella delivery mechanism is built on a 6 F catheter with locking tip, which interlocks with the central hub of the device. The entire system is threaded over a guide wire. Withdrawal of the guide wire after implantation of the device will unlock the mechanism, thereby disconnecting the umbrella from the delivery system. The umbrella collapsed into a pod, the centering mechanism folded and the delivery system can all be loaded into a 14 or 16 F long sheath. The umbrellas were manufactured in three sizes: 25, 30 and 35 mm. An umbrella that is approximately twice the stretched size of the ASD is chosen for implantation. First, the tip of the pod containing the umbrella is advanced into the left-atrium through the ASD (Figure 2 a). Then, the umbrella and centering mechanism delivered into the mid left atrium by retracting the tip of the sheath or pod (Figure 2 b). The entire system is then slowly withdrawn. The centering mechanism keeps the umbrella centered over the ASD. Further withdrawal results in embedding the hooks of the umbrella onto the left atrial side of the atrial septum (Figure 2 c). After the umbrella is fixed to the atrial septum, the umbrella delivery system is disconnected and removed. Experimental studies in closing surgically created ASDs in dogs and calves have indicated the feasibility of the method with excellent endothelialization of the umbrella components (Rashkind, 1975).

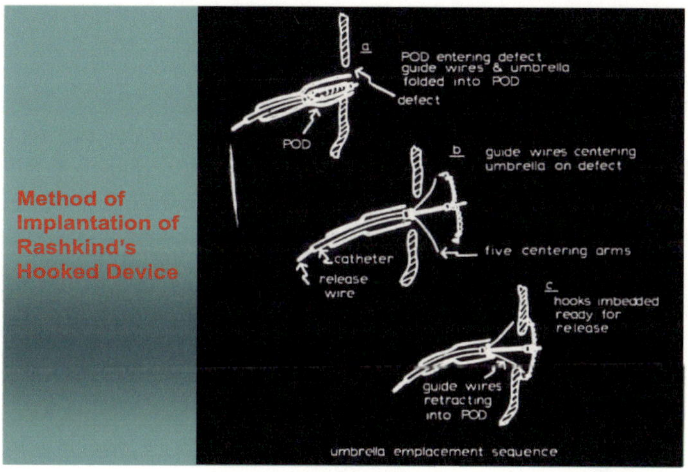

Fig. 2. Sequence of hooked prosthesis implantation (see text for details).

The senior author had the privilege of spending a month-long mini-sabbatical with Dr. William Rashkind in mid-1979 and during that period, had the opportunity in performing ASD device closures with the hooked device, both in calf model and in patients under the direction of Rashkind. Rashkind's enthusiasm and dedication in developing transcatheter closure methodology is laudable and the diligence with which he pursued the project is admirable. Subsequently, Rashkind obtained investigational device exemption from the FDA and began organizing multi-institutional clinical trials in the US in early 1980s. This is probably the first clinical trial for device implantation in pediatric cardiac practice. Unfortunately, Rashkind did not live to witness the conclusion of these trials or to see the monumental effect that his work had on the evolution of transcatheter occlusion technology.

Following experimental studies in animal models, Rashkind studied ASD closure in human subjects (Rashkind, 1983; Rashkind & Cuaso, 1977). A total of 33 patients were recruited for the clinical trial. Device implantation was not attempted in 10 patients because the defect was too large (N=6) to safely implant the device or too small (N=4) to warrant the potential risk of device placement. In the remaining 23 patients, 14 (61%) had adequate ASD closure and in nine (39%) the results were considered unsatisfactory. The initial six device implantations were three-rib umbrellas and the remaining were six-rib prostheses. Urgent surgical intervention was required in some patients to address the unsatisfactory implantations and others underwent elective surgery. However, uneventful surgical closure of the ASD and removal of the device were undertaken in all subjects. Clinical application in a limited number of patients by Beekman et al (1989) showed similar results.

Although good results were achieved in >50% patients, a number of problems were identified: requirement of a large sheath for implantation, uncertainty of whether the tissue will bind to the entire rim of the single disc device and difficulty in disengaging and repositioning the device if the hooks of the umbrella accidentally engage onto the left atrial wall or mitral valve. Because of these reasons, Rashkind modified this device into a double disc prosthesis which he had successfully employed to close an ASD in a cow (Rashkind, 1983). This modification was patterned after a concurrently developed Rashkind's patent ductus arteriosus occluding device (Rashkind, 1983; Rashkind et al., 1987).

2.3 Transformation from Rashkind to clamshell

The double-umbrella Rashkind device was subsequently utilized in closing ASDs by other workers (Lock et al., 1987, 1989; Rome et al., 1990). Whilst the results appeared good, difficulty in delivering umbrellas on either side of the defect, centering the device because of the angle of the delivery catheter (Lock et al., 1987) and inability of the umbrellas to fold back against each other, the device was modified by introducing a second spring in center of the arms (Lock et al., 1989) and was named Lock Clamshell Occluder. The clamshell device was initially used to occlude experimentally created ASDs in lambs: successful implantation was accomplished in six of the eight lambs. Embolization occurred in the remaining two. Complete occlusion of the ASD was noted in four lambs. Endothelialization of the device components was demonstrated in two lambs followed for 1 and 2 months after device deployment.

The clamshell device is composed of two opposing umbrellas made of 4 steel arms covered with woven Dacron material (Figure 1C). The steel arms are hinged together in the center of the device and the springs in the middle of the arm were introduced to facilitate folding back of the umbrellas against each other, thereby creating a clamshell configuration. The device is delivered through an 11 F sheath, a definitive improvement compared to the sheath size required to implant King's and hooked Rashkind's devices. Several device sizes were manufactured: 17 mm, 23 mm, 28 mm and 33 mm. Balloon stretched diameter of the ASD was measured as in the previous device implantation reports and a device at least 1.6 times larger than stretched ASD diameter was recommended for device placement. The delivery catheter is advanced into the left atrium across the ASD, and its tip positioned in mid-left atrium. The distal arms of the device are opened and the device is withdrawn against the atrial septum until the arms are seen to bend. The sheath is pulled back while keeping the device in position with resultant opening of the proximal arms in the right atrium. After ensuring the stability of the device across the atrial septum by fluoroscopic and echocardiographic imaging, the device is released by activating pin-to-pin mechanism.

The preliminary clinical experience included 17 clamshell device implantations (Rome et al., 1990). This report (Rome et al., 1990) combines the results of implantation of Rashkind double umbrella, prototype clamshell and clamshell devices and therefore the exact clamshell results are difficult to discern. Forty patients were taken to catheterization laboratory with intent to close, and of these, 34 (85%) had implantation of the device. With the exception of one major complication (death secondary to cerebral embolus, presumably related to dislodgment of iliac vein thrombus during placement of device delivery sheath), the procedures were successful. Embolization of the device into the descending aorta at iliac bifurcation occurred in two (6%) patients. The embolized devices were transcatheter retrieved and the patients sent to elective closure of their ASDs. At short-term follow-up, 12 (63%) of 19 who had adequate echocardiographic study had no residual shunts.

Hellenbrand et al reported use of this device; device implantation was attempted in eleven patients aged 13 months to 46 years (Hellenbrand et al., 1990). The device was implanted successfully in ten patients; the single failure was in their youngest patient weighing 11 kg. The procedures were performed under general anesthesia with endotracheal intubation and transesophageal echo-Doppler (TEE) monitoring; they advocated TEE monitoring during the procedure. Residual shunt was present in one (10%) patient. In the study by Boutin et al (1993), residual shunt was present in 91% immediately following device placement. The residual shunts decreased to 53% at a mean follow-up of 10 months. Actuarial analysis indicated progressive reduction of shunt with time (Boutin et al., 1993). Clinical trials by these and other investigators continued (Boutin et al., 1993; Latson, 1993; Perry et al., 1993). However, fractures of the arms of the device were reported in 40 to 84% of implanted devices with occasional embolization (Justo et al., 1996; Perry et al., 1993; Prieto et al., 1996), which were of concern. Consequently, further clinical trials with the device were suspended in 1991 by the investigators and the FDA. Subsequently the device was modified which will be reviewed later in this chapter.

2.4 Buttoned device

Sideris et al described "buttoned device" at about the time of transformation of Rashkind double disk device to clamshell device (Sideris et al., 1990 a & b). The device consisted of three components: occluder, counter-occluder and delivery system. The occluder consisted of an x-shaped, Teflon-coated wire skeleton covered with 1/8-in polyurethane foam (Figure 1 D, left component). The wire skeleton of the occluder can be folded, making the wires parallel, which can then be introduced into an 8-French sheath. When delivered to site of implantation, the occluder springs opens into its original square-shaped structure. A 2-mm string loop made of silk thread is attached to the center of the occluder; the loop is closed with a 1-mm knot (button). The counter-occluder is composed of a single strand, Teflon-coated wire skeleton covered with rhomboid shaped polyurethane foam (Figure 1 D, right component). A rubber piece is sutured in its center and becomes a buttonhole. The delivery system consisted of a) Teflon-coated 0.035-in guide wire (loading wire), b) a folded 0.008-in nylon thread passing through the guide wire, after having its core removed. The loop of this thread passes through the loop in the center of the occluder, c) an 8-French or 9-French long sheath for device delivery and implantation and d) an 8-French pusher catheter to advance the occluder and counter occluder within the sheath. This may be considered first generation buttoned device. The device was manufactured in 5-mm increments beginning with 25-mm size. The device size was measured by the diagonal length of the occluder and is same as the length of the counter-occluder.

Atrial septal defects were produced in piglets. The buttoned device was successfully implanted in 17 (85%) of 20 attempts. The failures were in the first three animals; presumably related inexperience of the operator and design imperfections (Sideris et al., 1990a). Full occlusion of the ASD and endothelialization of the device was demonstrated in all the 17 successful implantations.

During the preliminary clinical experience with this device (Rao et al., 1992a), minutes after implantation of the device, it spontaneously dislodged from the ASD site in one child. Inspection of the surgically explanted device revealed that the tie binding the occluder with the counter-occluder was torn. It seemed that excessive force was used while buttoning the components of the device across the atrial septum, to ensure adequate buttoning. Based on this undesirable experience, the device was modified by a) strengthening the button-loop by replacing the silk tie with 4-lb proof nylon, b) introducing a radio-opaque marker on the button, so that passage of the buttonhole of the counter-occluder over the button can be visualized by fluoroscopy. Consequently, there will be no need to use excessive force and c) the 1/8-in polyurethane foam covering the wire skeleton was replaced with thinner 1/16-in foam. This is considered second-generation of the buttoned device (Figure 3, left).

While incorporation of radio-opacity in the button made easy visualization of the button (Figure 4), it produced eccentricity of the button (Figure 3, left). This created additional difficulty in buttoning. Therefore, an additional loop of nylon thread was added immediately below the button (Figure 3, middle). This transformed the eccentric button of the second-generation device to be aligned straight, thus making it easier to button the occluder and counter-occluder across the atrial septum; this became third-generation device. Although the prevalence of unbuttoning decreased with the introduction of the additional loop (Rao et al,. 1994), buttoning across a thick atrial septum, especially when closing patent foramen ovale for prevention of presumed paradoxical embolism (Ende et al., 1996), became difficult with the radio-opaque wire of the counter-occluder swayed away from radio-opaque button despite "adequate buttoning." This, along with our experience with buttoned device for patent ductus arteriosus (Rao et al., 1993) in which we used two knots (buttons), the device was further modified such that an 8-mm string loop is attached to the occluder with two knots (buttons) on it, 4-mm and 8-mm from the occluder (Figure 3, right). Radio-opaque spring buttons were incorporated into both the knots. A sketch with details of the button loop and photographs of the fourth generation device are shown in figures 5 and 6, respectively.

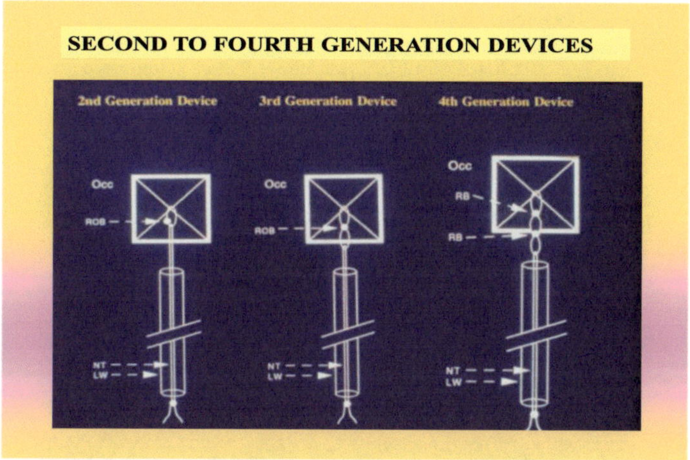

Fig. 3. Second, third and fourth generation buttoned devices; see the text for details. Occ, occluder; ROB, Radio-opaque button, NT, nylon thread; LW, loading wire.

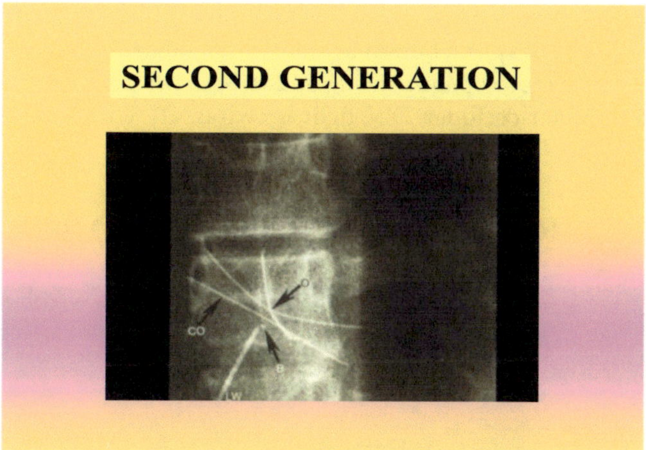

Fig. 4. Selected cinefluorograms in AP view demonstration the buttoning: the occluder (O) and the counter-occluder (CO) are past the radio-opaque button (B). LW, loading wire.

During the initial period of the clinical trials the device delivery required cutting the valve component of the delivery sheath which was then re-attached after loading the device into the sheath (Sideris et al., 1990b; Rao et al., 1991; Rao et al., 1992 a & b). This step was subsequently eliminated by directly loading the device into a short sheath which was then introduced thru' the valve of the delivery sheath (Rao, 2003). During this period the device was directly delivered across the defect. In cases with misplacement or slippage of the occluder into the right atrium, it was difficult to reposition the occluder and it had to be retrieved out of the patient, damaging the device. Therefore, over-the-wire delivery technique was developed. The implantation of the device is similar to direct delivery except the central foam part (close to middle of the X) is pierced with the end of 025" Amplatz wire and the wire is removed at the end of the procedure. The majority of devices were delivered by the over-the-wire technique in the later part of fourth generation device trials (Rao & Sideris, 1998; Rao et al., 2000; Rao, 2003).

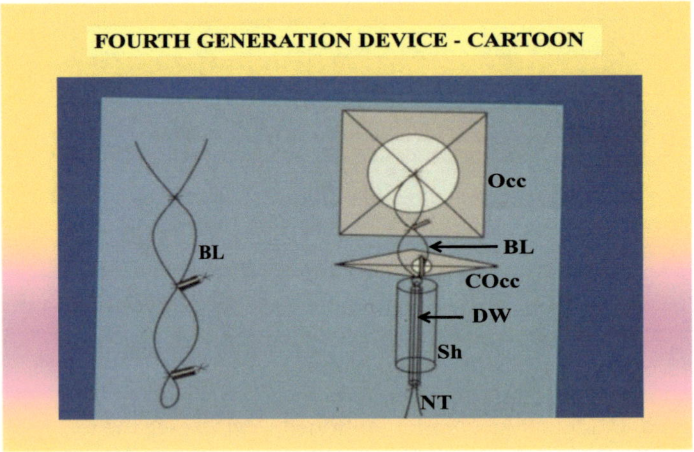

Fig. 5. Cartoon of the fourth generation buttoned device (right) with details of the buttoned loop (BL) (left). The buttoned loop (BL) includes two "spring" buttons positioned 4-mm apart. During buttoning, the spring button becomes straightened in line with the button loop. After buttoning the radio-opaque spring button becomes perpendicular, preventing unbuttoning. COcc, counter-occluder; DW, delivery wire; NT, nylon thread; Occ, occluder; Sh, sheath.

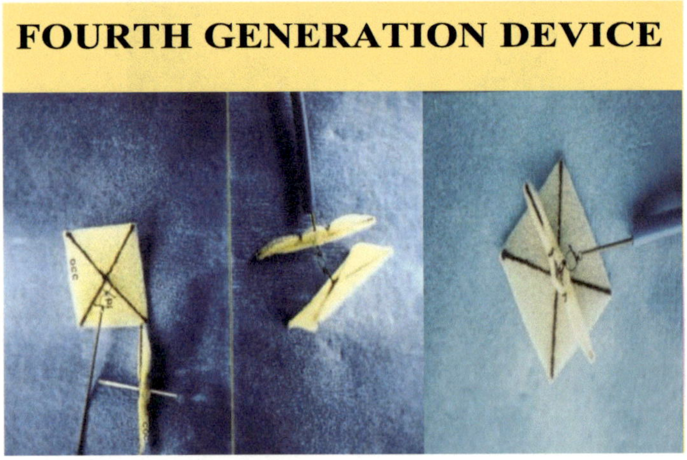

Fig. 6. Photographs of fourth generation buttoned device in multiple views.

Concomitantly a number of other modifications of the device were introduced which include, centering device (Sideris et al., 1996) to center the device over the defect (Figure 7), inverted device (Rao et al. 1997;) to address closure of right to left shunts (Figure 8), centering on demand device (Sideris et al., 1997; Rao & Sideris 2001) to center the device when necessary (Figure 9) and hybrid device (Rao, 2003) to address closure of defects with associated with atrial septal aneurysm (Figure 10).

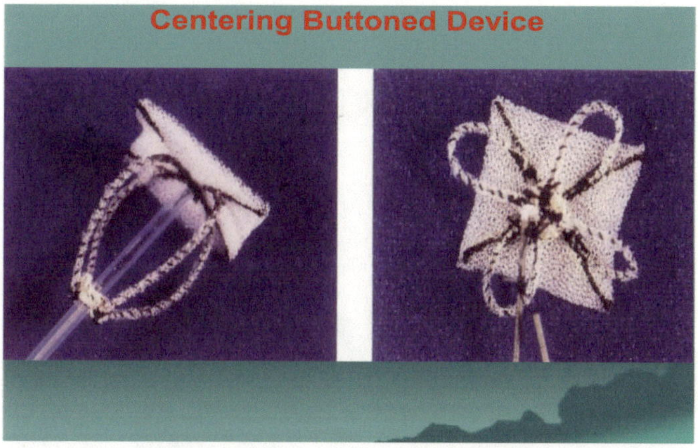

Fig. 7. Photographs of centering buttoned device with the centering mechanism open (left panel) and closed (right panel).

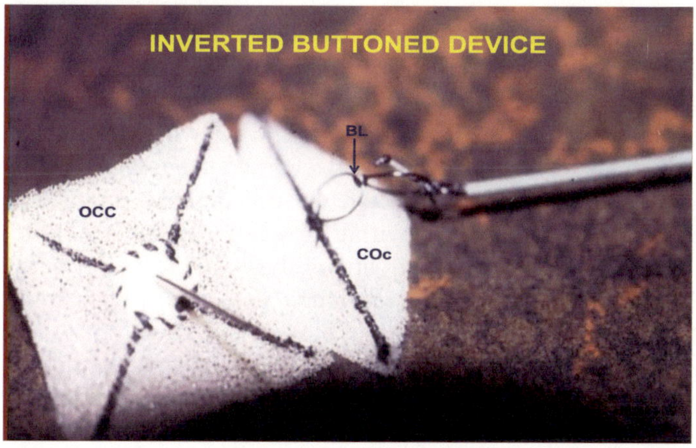

Fig. 8. Photograph of inverted buttoned device. COc, counter occluder; OCC, Occluder.

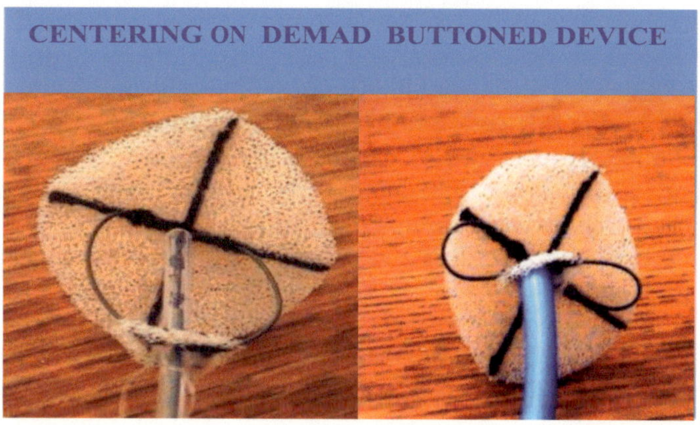

Fig. 9. Photographs of centering on demand buttoned device with the centering mechanism open (left panel) and closed (right panel).

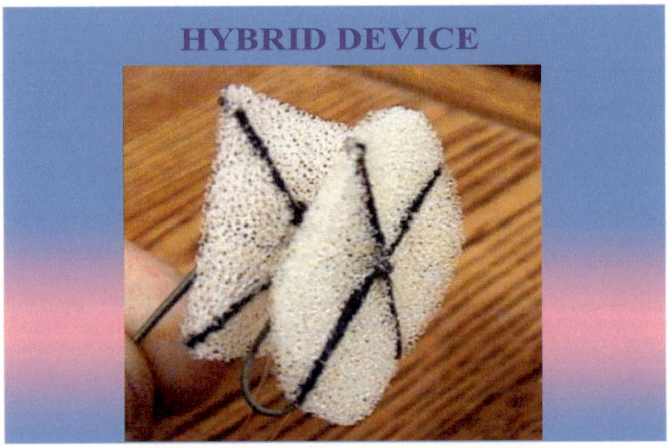

Fig. 10. Photograph of a hybrid device with square-shaped counter occluder on the aright atrial side, particular usefully with ASDs with atrial septal aneurysms.

A comprehensive review and comparison from international and US trials of the first four generations of buttoned device and the COD device was presented in 2001 (Rao and Sideris, 2001). The first three generation devices were used during a 3.5-year period ending in February 1993 in 180 patients at 16 institutions around the world (Rao et al., 1994). The ASD size varied between 5 and 25 mm. The device size varied between 25 and 50 mm. Successful implantation rate was 92% (166/180). Effective closure, defined as no (92 patients) or trivial (62 patients) shunt by echocardiography within 24 hours was achieved in 154 patients (92%). Unbuttoning occurred in 13 patients (7.2%) and of these, 10 (5.5%) had surgical retrieval and closure of their ASD. In a 7 -year follow-up study (Rao at al. 2000), residual shunts were closed surgically in 13 and by catheter methodology in 1 patient. In the remaining patients, the shunt either disappeared or decreased. The fourth generation device was implanted during a 4-year period ending in September 1997 in 423 patients at 40 institutions worldwide (Rao et al., 2000). The ASD size varied between 5 and 30 mm (median 17 mm). The device size varied between 25 and 60 mm and the successful implantation rate was 99.8% (422/423). Unbuttoning diminished to 0.9% and device embolization occurred in only one patient. Four patients had device retrieval and subsequent surgical repair and one patient required urgent surgical retrieval and ASD repair. Effective closure, as previously defined, was 90% (377 /417). Follow-up data were available up to a 5-year period in 333 of 417 patients (80%). During this period re-intervention occurred in 21 patients (5%) mainly due to residual shunts. This included 11 patients requiring surgical closure and 9 patients receiving a second device. In the remaining patients, there was a gradual reduction in residual shunt. The COD device was implanted in 65 of 68 patients (95.6%) during an 18 month period ending in July 2000 (Rao and Sideris, 2001). In the remaining 3 patients, the device was not implanted either because of a large defect with deficient rims (n = 1) or because the device was unstable (n = 2). In the latter two patients, the device was transcatheter retrieved, and all three patients underwent successful surgical closure electively. Based on echo-Doppler studies performed within 24 hours of device implantation, effective occlusion defined as no (n = 45; 69%) or trivial (n = 17; 26%) shunt was seen in 62 (95.4%) of 65 patients. In the remaining three, residual shunts were small and were followed-up clinically. One pediatric patient had a suspected thrombus on the occluder disc, which was treated with tissue plasminogen activator (tPA). The clot resolved without complications. At the time of that report (Rao and Sideris, 2001), short-term follow-up indicated that no further interventions had been required. An updated experience in 80 patients (Rao, 2003) indicated similar results.

The device has also been successfully used to close atrial defects presumed to be responsible for paradoxical embolism and cerebrovascular accidents (Ende et al., 1996), patent foramen ovale causing hypoxemia in platypnea-orthodeoxia syndrome in the elderly (Rao et al., 2001) and persistent right to left shunt associated with previously operated complex congenital cardiac anomalies, including Fontan fenestrations (Rao et al., 1997).

A number of single institutional (Sideris et al., 1990; Rao et al., 1991; Rao et al., 1992a; Rao et al., 1992b; Rao et al., 1995; Arora et al., 1996; Haddad et al., 1996; Worms et al., 1996) and multi-institutional (Rao et al., 1994; Lloyd et al., 1994; Zamora et al., 1998; Rao et al., 1998; Rao & Sideris et al., 1998; Rao et al., 2000; Rao and Sideris, 2001) clinical trials were undertaken which demonstrated feasibility, safety and effectiveness of this device. However, pre-market-approval (PMA) application was not made and consequently the device is not approved by the FDA and is not available for general clinical use.

2.5 Monodisk device

Pavcnik et al (Pavcnik et al., 1993) designed a monodisk device. The device consists of a stainless steel ring constructed with wire coil covered with two layers of nylon mesh. Three hollow pieces of braided stainless steel wires were sutured onto the right atrial side of the device (Figure 11). Three strands of monofilament nylon pass through, one in each of the hollow wires. The nylon thread also passes through the delivery catheter. The entire system

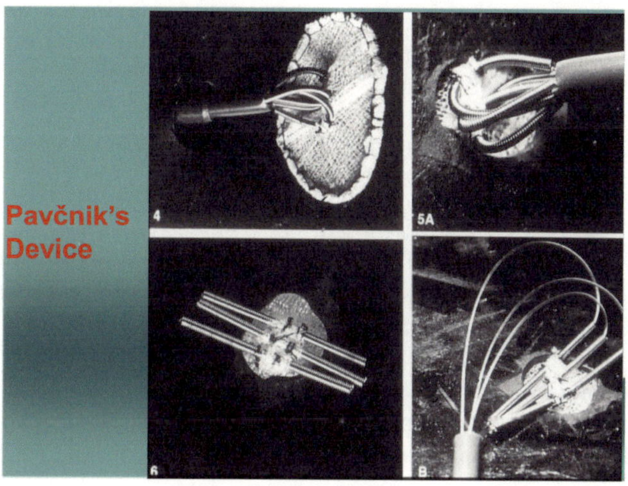

Fig. 11. Photographs of the monodisk device showing tilted side profile of the device after having opened it following passage through a model atrial septal defect (left top). Right atrial views of the device after having the device pulled against the model atrial septal defect prior to (right upper) and after (right lower) releasing flexible wires against the atrial septum are shown. Final position of the device (left lower) after disconnecting device by cutting monofilament nylon.

can be loaded and the device delivered through a 9 F sheath. Once the device is opened in the left atrium, it is withdrawn against the atrial septum so that the hollow wires are positioned onto the right atrial side of the septum (Figure 11, right upper panel). The nylon filaments are cut, which allow the wires to spring back and detach the device from the delivery catheter (Figure 11, right lower and left lower).

Device implantation to occlude five experimentally created ASDs in dogs was undertaken. The position of the device was good in all dogs and there was no residual shunt. In four dogs, postmortem studies were performed six months later, which showed the device to be in place with incorporation into the atrial septum and excellent endothelialization. The device was used successfully in two patients with secundum ASD (personal communication: D. Pavčnik, December 2000). More recently, a biodisk device was developed and animal experimentation suggested that device deployment is feasible, safe and effective (Pavčnik et al., 2010). The authors recommended long-term studies were to evaluate its long-term effectiveness.

2.6 Modified Rashkind PDA umbrella device

The Rashkind PDA umbrella (Rashkind et al., 1987) device was modified by bending the arms of the device such that there is a better apposition of the umbrellas against each other and the atrial septum (Redington & Rigby, 1994). The device was used to occlude four ASDs with left-to-right shunt. In two (50%) patients, the ASD was successfully closed. The remaining two (50%) patients required surgical removal of the device along with closure of the ASD. The device was also used to occlude 11 fenestrated Fontans. In nine patients, there was improvement in oxygen saturation. In the remaining two (18%), the procedure failed. To my knowledge, there are no other reports on the use of this modification by this or other workers. In addition, a similar bend placed in the clamshell device has resulted in breakage of the arms, forcing its removal from use. Therefore, advisability of introducing such a bend in the Rashkind PDA device was questioned (Rao & Sideris, 1995).

2.7 Atrial Septal Defect Occluding System (ASDOS)

Babic and his associates (Babic et al., 1991) described a double umbrella device implanted via arterio-venous guide wire loop in 1991. They named it ASDOS (atrial septal defect occluding system) (Sievert et al., 1995; 1998). In the initial prototype, once the device was locked in place, it required surgical removal for suboptimal positioning. The device underwent further modifications and the updated prototype was released in 1994. This version consists of two major components: (1) a prosthesis consisting of two self-opening umbrellas made of Nitinol wire frame and a thin membrane of polyurethane (Figure 12A) and (2) a delivery system. Each umbrella has five arms, which assume a round shape in the open position. When joined together, the umbrellas assume a discoid shape in profile and a "flower" shape in the frontal view. Umbrella sizes from 25 mm to 50 mm; with 5mm increments were manufactured. This system uses 11-F long sheath for device deployment.

Inter-atrial communications were created with dilatation balloons in 20 pigs and their defects closed with ASDOS device. Examination 3, 4 and 6 months after device closure revealed that devices were completely covered with smooth, scar-like tissue after three months of the procedure (Schneider et al., 1995; Thomsen-Bloch, 1995).

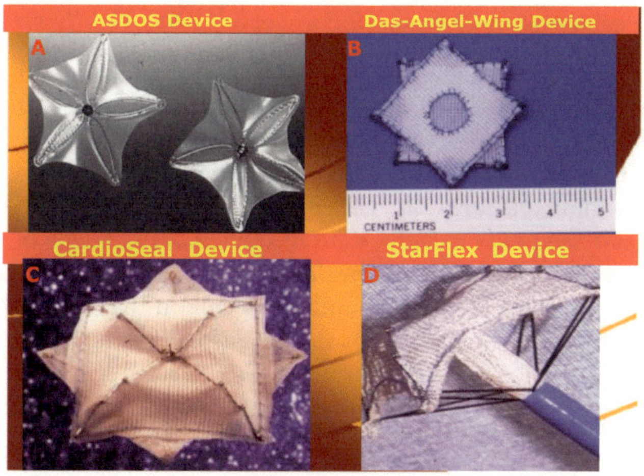

Fig. 12. Photographs of ASDOS (A), Das Angel Wing (B), CardioSEAL (C) and STARFlex (D) devices; see the text for detailed description of the devices.

Initial clinical trials in adult subjects (Babic et al., 1991; Sievert et al., 1995) and children (Hausdorf et al., 1996) demonstrated feasibility of the method and a multi-institutional clinical trial in 20 European institutions began (Sievert et al., 1998). Babic (Babic, 2000; Babic et al., 2003) reviewed the experience with the ASDOS system, including the European multi-institutional study. Between 1995 and 1998, closure was attempted in 350 patients (ASDOS registry, December 1998); 261 had ASDs and 89 had PFOs. It should be noted that 800 patients with ASD were screened and 261 (33%) of these were selected for device closure. Three hundred and eighteen patients (91%) had successful implantation. There were 32 (9%) failures; 26 devices were retrieved via catheter (7%) and 6 devices retrieved by surgery (2%). Early embolization was noted in 3 (0.9%), thromboemboli in 3 (0.9%), perforations in 6 (1.6%) and suspected infections in 2 (0.6%). Embolizations were to the right ventricular outflow tract, the abdominal aorta and the pulmonary artery. There were no late dislodgments or embolizations. Residual shunts were noted in 25% to 30% of patients and in some patients the shunt closed over time. A medium-to-large shunt remained in 8% and the defects were surgically repaired because of no shunt reduction with time. During follow-up, surgical extraction was performed in 11 (3%) patients. The complications include frame fractures in 20% of patients, thrombus formation in 25% patients and atrial wall perforation in 1.5% patients. Presumably because of these complications, the device was renounced by the inventor (Babic et al., 2003) and is not currently used. A modified version with a stent between the umbrellas to provide optimal centering along with other changes was conceived, but not available for clinical use (Babic et al. 2003).

2.8 Das Angel Wing Device

In 1993, Das and his colleagues (Das et al., 1993) designed a self-centering device, delivered transvenously via an 11 F sheath and named it Das Angel Wing Device (Figure 12B). This device had two polyester fabric-covered square frames and a Nitinol frame with midpoint torsion spring eyelets. A circular hole with a diameter equal to one-half of the size of the disk was punched from the right disk with the margins sewn to the left-sided disk forming a conjoined ring, the centering mechanism (Rickers et al., 1998). Device sizes ranging from 12 to 40 mm were manufactured. The length of the square of the device determines device size.

ASDs were produced surgically in 20 adult canines. Percutaneous closure was attempted in all and was successful in 19 (95%). Following closure, angiography revealed no shunts in 17 and trivial shunts in 2. Six dogs were followed for 2 to 8 months; trivial shunt present in 1 animal immediately after closure had closed by the time of the repeat study. Device embolization was not seen either at the time of device deployment or during follow-up. Microscopy at 8 weeks in 3 dogs showed the devices to be covered by smooth endocardium, enmeshed in mature collagen tissue. The authors conclude that this self-centering device, with effective and safe ASD closure in a canine model, supports its use in human clinical trials (Das et al., 1993).

Clinical trials were undertaken in US and abroad (Rickers et al., 1998; Banerjee et al., 1999). Phase I clinical trial included 90 patients; 50 of these were ostium secundum ASDs (Banerjee et al., 1999; Das et al., 2003). The ASD size varied between 2 and 20 mm. The device size varied between 18 and 35 mm. The device was successfully implanted in 46 (92%) patients; in the remaining four patients surgical retrieval of the mal-positioned device along with surgical closure of ASD was accomplished without additional complications. Significant procedure related complications were seen in three patients. Follow-up echo studies were available in 34 and in 31 of these, there was no residual shunt. A phase II trial involving 47 patients followed with essentially similar results as those of phase I trials (Das et al., 2003). Prior to the conclusion of phase II trial, the investigation was halted in attempts to reconfigure the device. The new device modification, Guardian Angel wing (Angel wing II) included rounded right and left atrial disks, to be easily retrievable, to be easily repositioned and to maintain the self-centering mechanism. Although it was stated that the re-made device will enter clinical trials in the near future (Das et al., 2003), to our knowledge, there has been no further activity reported of either the Angel Wing or Guardian Angel devices; it would appear that the device was shelved.

2.9 CardioSEAL and STARFlex devices

As mentioned in the previous section of this paper, following withdrawal of clamshell device because of breakage of arms (stress fractures), the device was redesigned by replacing stainless steel of the umbrella arms with MP35N, a nonferrous alloy and by introducing an additional bend in the arms of the device; the device was named CardioSEAL (Figure 12 C) in 1996 (Ryan et al., 1998). Subsequently the device was modified to introduce self-centering mechanism by attaching micro springs between the umbrellas, and is named STARFlex (Figure 12 D) in 1998 (Hausdorf et al., 1999).

Both CardioSEAL and STARFlex devices were used in the European multicenter trial (Carminati et al., 2000; Bennhagen et al., 2003) conducted from October 1996 to April 1999; device implantation was attempted in 334 patients with success in 325 (97.3%) patients. Device to balloon stretched ASD diameter ratio was 2.16 (mean). Embolization of the device occurred shortly after the procedure in 13 patients (4%); 12 embolized to the pulmonary artery and one to the left ventricle. In ten patients, surgical retrieval and ASD closure was performed while the remaining three had catheter retrieval with successful re-implantation of another device. One patient had hemiplegia four hours after the procedure. A residual shunt was present in

41% immediately following the procedure, which decreased to 31% at time of discharge and to 21% six and 12 months later. During follow-up surgery was required in two more patients and wire frame fractures were observed in 6.1% patients. The authors concludes that these devices are useful to close small to moderate ASDs and when used to close large defects, complications or less than optimal results are likely. Similar results were reported in the Canadian experience with CardioSEAL device in 50 patients (Pedra et al., 2000).

STARFlex was further modified by replacing Dacron with bio-absorbable materials: BioSTAR and BioTREK; these devices will be discussed in a latter section of this paper.

2.10 Amplatzer septal occluder

In 1997, a new self-expanding Nitinol prosthesis was developed by Dr. Kurt Amplatz, which consists of two self-expandable round disks connected to each other with a short connecting waist (Sharafuddin et al., 1997) and is commonly referred to as Amplatzer septal occluder (Figure 13 A). Nitinol is a nickel-titanium compound consisting of 55% nickel and 45% titanium and has a property of resuming the original shape (shape memory) when deployed. The device size is determined by the waist diameter and ranges from 4 to 40 mm. The disk diameters increase with increasing waist diameters.

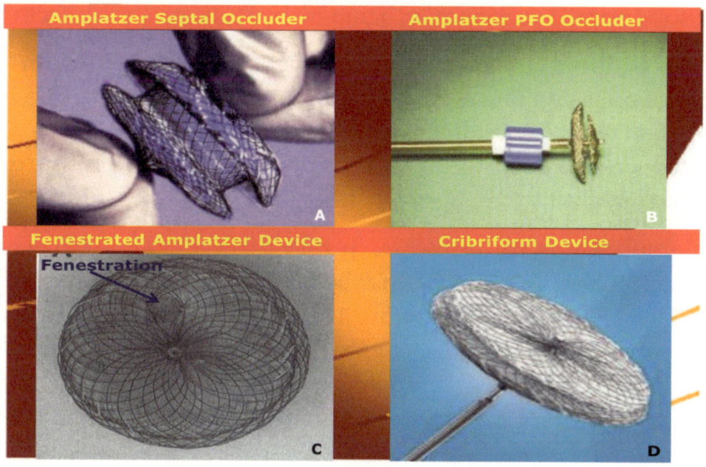

Fig. 13. Photographs of Amplatzer septal occluder (A), PFO Occluder (B), fenestrated Amplatzer device (C) and cribriform Amplatzer device (D).

ASDs were created surgically in 15 mini-pigs; the ASD diameter ranged between 10 and 16 mm. Amplatzer septal occluder was used to percutaneously close the ASDs (Sharafuddin et al., 1997). Successful implantation of the device was accomplished in 12 (80%) animals. Angiography revealed complete closure of ASD in 7 of 12 animals immediately after device placement and in 11 of 12 one week later. Fibrous incorporation of the device with neoendothelialization was seen within 3 months. The authors concluded that occlusion of secundum ASDs is feasible with this new device.

The device has been used widely in PFOs, ASDs, and Fontan fenestrations. The results of first clinical trial were reported by Masura in 1997 (Masura et al., 1997). The device was approved by FDA in December 2001 and has since been used extensively worldwide.

Detailed description of the device, implantation procedure and results were described in Chapter 1 and several other chapters in this book and will not be further discussed. Several modifications of the Amplatzer device were introduced: 1. PFO Occluder (Figure 13 B) to close patent foramen ovale (Han et al., 1999), 2. fenestrated Amplatzer device (Figure 13 C) to keep atrial septal defects or Fontan fenestration open to maintain cardiac output (Amin et al., 2002), restrict the size of defect to reduce the atrial shunt (Holtzer et al., 2005) or to serve as pop-off mechanism in severe pulmonary hypertension (Lammers et al., 2007), 3. cribriform device (Figure 13 D) to occlude multiple or fenestrated ASDs (Hijazi et al 2003) and 4. nanoplatinum coating to prevents nickel release from Amplatzer devices (Lertsapcharoen, 2008), thus preventing Kounis syndrome.

2.11 HELEX septal occluder

The HELEX septal occluder is made up of a single length of 0.012-in diameter Nitinol wire covered by an ultra thin membrane of ePTFE. The configuration, once delivered to the site of implantation, was two round and flexible disks (Figure 14 A), one on either side of the ASD. During delivery, the flexible frame is elongated around a central mandrel and fits through a 9F sheath. The wire mandrel except for the central locking mechanism is covered with ePTFE membrane so that only a small portion of Nitinol wire is exposed in the vascular system. Several sizes from 15 to 35 mm, in 5 mm increments were manufactured.

Device closure was performed in 24 dogs with surgically created ASDs with 100% successful implantation. Initial occlusion rate of 88% was found by transesophageal echocardiography which improved to 100% at 2-week follow-up (Zahn et al., 1999; 2001). These animal studies also demonstrated coverage of the defect components with fibrous connective tissue followed by neo-endothelialization, usually within three months.

The first clinical implant was performed by in 1999 (Latson et al., 2000), and the Food and Drug Administration phase I feasibility trial began in 2000. Feasibility study involving 63 patients, multicenter pivotal study including 143 subjects and continued access study that enrolled 156 patients (Feldman, 2010) demonstrated feasibility, safety and effectiveness of the device. The HELEX occluder was approved by FDA in 2006 and from then on it has been used extensively worldwide for closing small to medium sized ASDs and PFOs.

2.12 Sideris' Wire-less devices including transcatheter patch

Majority of ASD-occluding devices are double disc devices with wire components and have limitations. The major disadvantages are requirement of sufficient septal rims to hold the device in place and complications related to wire components (wire fractures and perforations) of the device. To address these problems, Sideris and colleagues developed wireless, transcatheter-implantable devices to occlude large ASDs (Sideris et al., 1999 a & b; Zamora et al., 2000; Sideris, 2003). Two devices were developed (Sideris, 2003): detachable balloon device and the transcatheter patch (Figure 14 B).

The detachable balloon device (DBD) consisted of balloon occluder, made from Latex in different sizes and a floppy disk, similar to the counter occluder described in the buttoned device section above. The DBDs were used to occlude of experimentally created ASDs in 20 piglets (Sideris et al., 2000a); in three experiments detachable double balloon devices were used. One device embolized into the descending aorta and complete occlusion was noticed in remaining pigs. Follow-up studies revealed that the detachable balloons lost their content and became flat in approximately two months and the device was covered by endothelial tissue in 3 to 4 weeks. Human feasibility study (Sideris et al., 1999a) involved six ostium secundum ASDs (among others); one device embolized, one patient had residual shunt which increased over time and four had good occlusion.

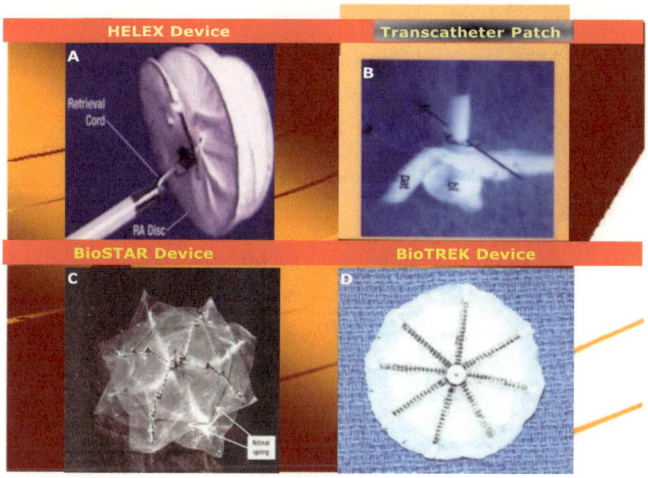

Fig. 14. Photographs of HELEX device (A), transcatheter patch (B), BioSTAR device (C) and BioTREK device (D).

The transcatheter patch device consisted of a flat or sleeve patch, a balloon support catheter and a safety thread; the patch, made up of polyurethane foam, covers the distal balloon. The occluding distal balloon (balloon/patch) is inflated at volumes 2 mm larger than the test-occluding diameter of the defect and held in place. The balloons were deflated and removed 48 hours later. This device was also tried in 20 experimentally created ASDs (Sideris et al., 2000b); ten were flat patches and ten sleeve patches. The patches were supported by balloon catheters from one to six days. Good occlusion of ASDs was seen if the supporting catheter was withdrawn 48 hours or later. Histological studies revealed formation fibrin and inflammatory cells. The sleeve patch appeared to be better centered over the defect than a flat patch. Initial clinical trials were performed in a limited number of patients (Sideris, 2003). Subsequently (Sideris et al., 2010), a larger number (N=74) of patients participated in the clinical trial. The age of the subjects varied from 1.5 to 67 years and their defect sizes were from 13 to 35 mm (mean=25) in diameter; 88% had effective occlusion immediately after deployment of the patch which increased to 96% at follow-up (Sideris et al., 2010).

Initially, this device required keeping the balloon in place up to 48 hours to allow the patch to adhere to the septal wall, an obvious disadvantage of this technique (King & Mills, 2010). To address this problem, Sideris et al (2010) developed accelerated release technique by applying polyethylene glycol-based surgical adhesive to the surface of the patch immediately prior to its implantation. This method was used in 9 patients with ASD diameters ranging from six and 25 mm. Effective occlusion immediately after implantation occurred in 78% which improved to 100% a follow-up. An immediate release patch (IRP) was developed which uses a single latex balloon, a safety bioabsorbable thread (Vicryl, Ethicon, a Johnson & Johnson company, Somerville, NJ) and polyurethane patch with surgical adhesive that was used in accelerated release technique. The addition of the adhesive makes the device release immediate and attachment to the septum (mediated by fibrin formation) takes place in approximately 48 hours (Sideris et al., 2010). The IRP was used in 10 subjects with defects ranging from 12 to 26 mm; 100% full occlusion both at implantation and at follow-up was reported (Sideris et al., 2010). Further clinical trials are planned.

2.13 New devices

Subsequent to the development of the devices reviewed in the preceding sections additional devices were designed and tested. None of these are approved by the FDA for routine clinical use and will be reviewed briefly.

These devices, to the best of our knowledge, are bio-absorbable NMT devices (Bio-STAR and Bio-TREK), Occlutech device, Cardia devices (INTRASEPT, ATRIASEPT I/II-ASD and ULTRASEPT), Solysafe Septal Occluder, pfm ASD-R device, Heart R Septal Occluder (manufactured in China) and others.

2.13.1 BioSTAR and BioTREK

When occluding devices are implanted to close ASDs, the left atrium is essentially inaccessible, should trans-septal intervention becomes necessary later in life such as mapping and ablation of left-sided accessory pathways, mitral valve interventions, left atrial appendage occlusion and others. To address this concern, NMT Medical Inc. (Boston, MA) modified the STARFlex device by replacing Dacron with heparin-coated, acellular, tissue engineered, porcine intestinal collagen matrix that allows absorption and replacement of the membrane with human tissue, and was named BioSTAR (Figure 14C). Studies in sheep model (Jux et al., 2003; 2006) demonstrated rapid endothelialization of the device and resorption of intestinal collagen matrix over a period of 2 years. Feasibility, safety, and effectiveness of closure of ASDs with BioSTAR both in adults (Mullen et al., 2006) and children (Hoehn et al., 2010) were demonstrated.

The supporting arms (ribs) of the BioSTAR device however, continue to be metallic and are not bio-absorbable. BioTREK device (Figure 14 D) was developed and designed to be 100% reabsorbable. The covering discs as well as support ribs are made up of poly-4-hydroxybutyrate. Over time, the patches and the connecting ribs disappear, leaving the fibrous septum. The device was reported in preclinical testing (Kramer, 2010). Other workers are developing additional biodegradable devices (Duong-Hong et al., 2010).

2.13.2 Occlutech

Occlutech septal occluder, initially designed to close PFOs (Krizanic et al. 2008) has been modified to close ASDs. The device is similar to Amplatzer in design (double-disc device composed of self-expanding Nitinol mesh wire), but with use of unique braiding technology; the amount of metal is reduced by 50%. In addition, the left atrial hub is removed. The devices were implanted in 29 patients with PFO and in 12 patients with ASD.

TEE studies showed a residual shunt in 11.2% after 60 days in patients with PFO and a left-to-right shunt in 9.1% of the remaining patients with ASD. After 180 days only 1 patient (3.7%) with PFO had a right-to-left shunt. No residual shunts were observed in the patients with ASD (Krizanic et al., 2010).

2.13.3 Cardia devices (INTRASEPT, ATRIASEPT I/II-ASD and ULTRASEPT)

PFO-Star device, consisting of Ivalon foam double umbrella was developed in late 1990s by Cardia Inc. (Eagan, MN) for percutaneous closure of PFOs (Braun et al., 2002; Schraeder et al, 2003). This device may be considered Generation I and was modified several times, addressing its deficiencies with resultant development of Generation II, Generation III, Generation IV (INTRASEPT), Generation V (ATRIASEPT I-ASD and ATRIASEPT II-ASD) and Generation VI (ULTRASEPT) devices (Turner & Forbes, 2010). Generation V and VI devices were designed to deal with ostium secundum ASDs. Clinical trials with ATRIASEPT I-ASD device (Stolt et al., 2010; Turner & Forbes, 2010) showed favorable early results. Clinical trials with ATRIASEPT II-ASD and ULTRASEPT devices are planned (Turner & Forbes, 2010).

2.13.4 Solysafe septal occluder

The Solysafe Septal Occluder device (Swissimplant AG, Solothurn, Switzerland), designed by Dr. Lazlo Solymar of Gothenburg, consists of two foldable polyester patches attached to eight cobalt-based alloy (Phynox) wires. The course of the wires through the patches enables the device to center itself within the defect. The maximum diameter is given by the distance of the wires that are fixed in the patches. Several sizes, 25 mm thru' 44 mm are manufactured (Ewert, 2010). Two clinical trials with 44 and 32 patients (Ewert et al., 2008, Kretschmar et al., 2010) respectively were reported with implantation rates of 87% and closure rate of 100% at six month follow-up. The worldwide experience with this device was said to approximate 1,400 patients (Ewert, 2010).

2.13.5 The pfm ASD-R device

The pfm ASD-R devices were made up of tightly woven single piece of Nitinol wire mesh without welding or hubs and in their final form have a double-disc configuration. Animal experimentation in pigs revealed complete endothelialization in three weeks without significant inflammatory reaction (Granja & Freudenthal, 2010). The initial clinical application in 23 patients demonstrated good results and a multi-institutional phase II clinical trial in Argentina is planned (Granja & Freudenthal, 2010).

2.13.6 Other devices

Other devices such as Cardi-O-Fix Septal Occluder, Heart R Septal Occluder, cocoon, Lifetech device (also called sears device), some manufactured in China and others that may have escaped detection by our literature search may be in development.

3. Closure of patent foramen ovale

Some cerebrovascular accidents and other systemic arterial emboli, especially in young subjects are presumed to be due to paradoxical embolism through an atrial defect, most frequently a patent foramen ovale (PFO). Closure of such atrial defects is an alternative option to life-long anticoagulation. Non-surgical transcatheter occlusion of such a defect was first reported with King's device in 1976 (Mills & King, 1976). Mills and King effectively occluded an atrial defect with a 25 mm device in a 17-year-old male who had a hemiperetic stroke secondary to paradoxical embolism. Subsequently, clamshell (Bridges et al., 1992) and buttoned (Rao et al., 1992 a & b; Chandar et al., 1996; Ende et al., 1996) devices have been used to successfully occlude PFOs presumed to be the site of paradoxical embolism.

In addition, some PFOs are considered to be the seat of right to left shunt causing hypoxemia as seen in platypnea-orthodeoxia syndrome. Right to left shunt thru' PFO can also occur in patients who were previously treated for complex congenital cardiac anomalies including Fontan fenestrations as well as in patients who had right ventricular infarction. Decompression (Caisson's) illness and migraine have also been attributed to right to left shunt across PFO.

Majority of the ASD devices described in the preceding sections, as and when they became available, have also been used to close PFOs to address the above listed conditions. Moreover, either the existing devices were modified to address the anatomic features of the foramen ovale or new devices were designed to specifically address the PFOs and these include, Amplatzer PFO occluder, Cardia devices (PFO-Star and several of its subsequent generations), Premere occluder, Coherex Flat stent, PFx Closure System (not a device but employs monopolar radio frequency energy to effect closure of a PFO by welding the tissues of the septum primum with the septum secundum), pfm PFO-R, Solysafe PFO occluder and others. Because of limitation in space and the intent to mainly address history of ASD device closure, no further discussion of PFOs will be included.

4. Summary and conclusion

In this chapter, historical aspects of transcatheter atrial septal occluding devices are reviewed. Since the initial description of an ASD closing devices by King, Rashkind and their associates, a large number of single disc and double disc devices have been designed

and tested in animal models followed by clinical trials in human subjects. Feasibility, safety and effectiveness have been demonstrated with most devices. However, design, redesign, testing and re-testing have been the typical path with most devices. Currently, only two devices are approved by the FDA in the US and these are: Amplatzer septal occluder and HELEX septal occluder. Several other devices are in development, some at the stage of animal experimentation and some in clinical trials in Europe or US. We will await for additional devices to be approved for general clinical use so that the practicing interventional cardiologist will have several devices at his/her disposal so that an appropriate device that suits best for a given patient and his/her defect. A brief review of historical aspects of PFO closure was also included.

5. References

[1] Amin, Z.; Danford, D. A.; Pedra, C. A. (2002). A new Amplatzer device to maintain patency of Fontan fenestrations and atrial septal defects. *Catheter Cardiovasc Interv*, Vol. 57, No. 2, pp. 246-251

[2] Arora, R.; Trehan, V. K.; Karla, G. S.; et al. (1996). Transcatheter closure of atrial septal defect using buttoned device: Indian experience. *Indian Heart J,* Vol. 48, No.2, pp. 145-149

[3] Babic, U. (2000). Experience with ASDOS for transcatheter closure of atrial septal defect and patent foramen ovale. *Curr Intervent Cardiol Rep,* Vol. 2, No. 2, pp. 177-183

[4] Babic, U. U.; Grujicic. S.; Popvic, Z.; et al. (1991). Double-umbrella device for transvenous closure of patent ductus arteriosus and atrial septal defect: first clinical experience. *J Intervent Cardiol, Vol.* 4, No. 4, pp. 283-294

[5] Babic, U.; Sievert, H.; Schneider, M.; Babic, M. (2003). ASDOS-Atrial Septal Defect Occluder System, In: *Catheter Based Devices for Treatment of Noncoronary Cardiovascular Disease in Adults and Children,* P. S. Rao, M. J. Kern (Eds.): 35-43, Lippincott, Williams & Wilkins, Philadelphia, PA, USA.

[6] Banerjee, A.; Bengur, A. R.; Li, J. S.; et al. (1999). Echocardiographic characteristics of successful deployment of the Das Angel Wings atrial septal defect closure device: initial multicenter experience in the United States. *Am J Cardiol, Vol.* 83, No. 8, pp. 1236-1241

[7] Beekman, R. H.; Rocchini, A. P.; Snider, A. R.; et al. (1989). Transcatheter atrial septal defect closure: preliminary experience with the Rashkind occluder device. *J Intervent Cardiol, Vol. 2, No.* 1, pp. 35-41

[8] Bennhagen, R. G.; McLaughlin, P., Benson, L. N. (2003). CARDIOSEAL AND STARFLEX DEVICES, In: *Catheter Based Devices for Treatment of Noncoronary Cardiovascular Disease in Adults and Children,* P. S. Rao & M. J. Kern (Eds.): 61-69, Lippincott, Williams & Wilkins, Philadelphia, PA, USA.

[9] Bigelow, W. G.; Lindsey, W. E. & Greenwood, W. F. (1950). Hypothermia, it's possible role in cardiac surgery. *Ann Surg,* Vol. 132, No. 5, pp. 849-866

[10] Boutin, C.; Musewe, N. N.; Smallhorn, J. F.; et al. (1993). Echocardiographic follow- up of atrial septal defect after catheter closure by double-umbrella device. *Circulation,* Vol. 88, No. 2, pp. 621-627

[11] Braun, M. U.; Fassbender, D.; Schoen, S. P.; et al. (2002). Transcatheter closure of patent foramen ovale in patients with cerebral ischemia. *J Am Coll Cardiol,* Vol. 39, No. 12, pp. 2019-2025

[12] Bridges, N. D.; Hellenbrand, W.; Latson, L.; et al. (1992). Transcatheter closure of patent foramen ovale after presumed paradoxical embolism. *Circulation,* Vol. 86, No. 6, pp. 1902-1908

[13] Carminati, M.; Giusti, S.; Hausdorf, G.; et al. (2000). A European multicentre experience using the CardioSEAL® and Starflex double umbrella devices to close interatrial communications holes within the oval fossa. Cardiol Young, Vol. 10, No. 5, pp. 519-526

[14] Chandar, J. S. ; Rao, P. S. ; Lloyd, T. R. ; et al. (1999). Atrial septal defect closure with 4th generation buttoned device: results of US multicenter FDA Phase II clinical trial (Abstract). *Circulation,* Vol. 100, Suppl - I-708

[15] Das, G. S.; Harrison, J. K. & O'Laughlin, M. P. (2003). The Angel Wings Das device. In: *Catheter based devices for the treatment of non-coronary cardiovascular disease in adults and children.* P. S. Rao & M. J. Kern (Eds): 45-49, Lippincott Williams & Wilkins, Philadelphia, PA, USA

[16] Das, G. S.; Voss, G.; Jarvis, G.; et al. (1993). Experimental atrial septal defect closure with a new, transcatheter, self-centering device. *Circulation, Vol.* 88, No. 4, pp. 1754-1764
[17] Duong-Hong, D.; Tang, Y. D. & Wu, W. (2010). Fully biodegradable septal defect occluder-a double umbrella design. *Catheter Cardiovasc Interv,* Vol. 76, No. 5, pp. 711-718
[18] Ende, D. J.; Chopra, P. S. & Rao, P. S. (1996). Prevention of recurrence of paradoxic embolism: mid-term follow-up after transcatheter closure of atrial defects with buttoned device. *Am J Cardiol, Vol.* 78, No. 2, pp. 233-236
[19] Ewert, P. (2010). The Solysafe septal occluder for the closure of ASDs and PFOs. In: *Transcatheter closure of ASDs and PFOs: A comprehensive assessment,* Z. M. Hijazi, T. Feldman, M. H. Abdullah A Al-Qbandi, & H. Sievert (Eds): 417-422, Cardiotext, Minneapolis, MN, USA
[20] Ewert, P.; Soderberg, B.; Dahnert, I.; et al. (2008). ASD and PFO closure with the Solysafe septal occluder-Results of a prospective multicenter pilot study. *Cathet Cardiovasc Intervent,* Vol. 71, No. 3, pp. 398-402
[21] Feldman, T. (2010). The GORE HELEX septal occluder. In: *Transcatheter closure of ASDs and PFOs: A comprehensive assessment,* Z. M. Hijazi, T. Feldman, M. H. Abdullah A Al-Qbandi, & H. Sievert (Eds): 355-368, Cardiotext, Minneapolis, MN, USA
[22] Galal, M. O.; Wobst, A.; Halees, Z.; et al. (1994). Perioperative complications following surgical closure of atrial septal defect type II in 232 patients - a baseline study. *Europ Heart J,* Vol. 15, No. 10, pp. 1381-1384
[23] Gibbon, J. H., Jr. (1953) Application of a mechanical heart and lung apparatus to cardiac surgery. In: *Recent Advances in Cardiovascular Physiology and Surgery,* J. H. Gibbon, Jr (ed): 107-113, University of Minnesota, Minneapolis, MN, USA
[24] Granja, M. & Freudenthal, F. (2010). The pfm device for ASD closure. In: *Transcatheter closure of ASDs and PFOs: A comprehensive assessment.* Z. M Hijazi, T. Feldman, M. H. Abdullah A Al-Qbandi, & H. Sievert (Eds): 423-429, Cardiotext, Minneapolis, MN, USA
[25] Haddad, J.; Secches, A.; Finzi, L.; et al. (1996). Atrial septal defect: percutaneous transvenous occlusion with the buttoned device. *Arq Bras Cardiol,* Vol. 67, No. 1, pp. 17-22
[26] Han, Y. ; Gu, X. ; Titus, J. L. ; et al. (1999). New self-expanding patent foramen ovale occlusion device. *Cathet Cardiovasc Intervent,* Vol. 47, No. 3, pp. 370-376
[27] Holzer, R.; Cao, Q. L. & Hijazi, Z. M. (2005). Closure of a moderately large atrial septal defect with a self-fabricated fenestrated Amplatzer septal occluder in an 85- year-old patient with reduced diastolic elasticity of the left ventricle. *Catheter Cardiovasc Interv,* Vol. 64, No. 4, pp. 513-518
[28] Hausdorf, G.; Kaulitz. R. & Paul T. (1999). Transcatheter closure of atrial septal defect with a new flexible, self-centering device, The Starflex Occluder. *Am Heart J,* Vol. 84, No. 9, pp. 1113-1116
[29] Hausdorf, G.; Schneider, M.; Franzbach, B.; et al. (1996). Transcatheter closure of secundum atrial septal defects with the atrial septal defect occlusion system (ASDOS): initial experience in children. Heart, Vol. 75, No. 1, pp. 83-88
[30] Hellenbrand, W. E.; Fahey, J. T.; McGowan, F. X.; et al. (1990). Transesophageal echocardiographic guidance of transcatheter closure of atrial septal defect. *Am J Cardiol,* Vol. 66, No. 2, pp. 207-213

[31] Hijazi, Z. M. & Cao, Q-L. (2003). Transcatheter closure of multi-fenestrated atrial septal defects using the new Amplatzer cribriform device. *Congenital Cardiology Today*, Vol. 1, No. 1, pp. 1-4

[32] Hoehn, R.; Hesse, C.; Ince, H. & Peuster, M. (2010). First experience with the BioSTAR-device for various applications in pediatric patients with congenital heart disease. *Catheter Cardiovasc Interv*, Vol. 75, No. 1, pp. 72-77

[33] Justo, R. N.; Nykanen, D. G.; Boutin, C.; et al. (1996). Clinical impact of transcatheter closure of secundum atrial septal defects with double umbrella device. *Am J Cardiol*, Vol. 77, No. 10, pp. 889-892

[34] Jux, C.; Bertram, H.; Wohlsein, P.; et al. (2006). Interventional atrial septal defect closure using a totally bioresorbable occluder matrix: development and preclinical evaluation of the BioSTAR device. *J Amer Coll Cardiol*, Vol. 48, No. 1, pp. 161-169

[35] Jux, C.; Wohlsein, P.; Bruegmann, M.; et al. (2003). A new biological matrix for septal occlusion. *J Interv Cardiol*, Vol. 16, No. 2, pp. 149-52

[36] King, T. D. & Mills, N. L. (1974). Nonoperative closure of atrial septal defects. *Surgery*, Vol. 75, No. 3, pp. 383-388

[37] King, T. D.; Thompson, S. L.; Steiner, C.; et al. (1976). Secundum atrial septal defect: nonoperative closure during cardiac catheterization. *J Am Med Assoc, Vol.* 235, No. 25, pp. 2506-2509

[38] King, T. D.; Thompson, S. L.; Steiner, C.; et al. (1978). Measurement of atrial septal defect during cardiac catheterization: experimental and clinical trials. *Am J Cardiol*, Vol. 41, No. 3, pp. 537-542

[39] King, T. D & Mills, N. L. (2010). Historical perspectives on ASD device closure. In: *Transcatheter closure of ASDs and PFOs: A comprehensive assessment*, Z. M. Hijazi, T. Feldman, M. H. Abdullah A Al-Qbandi, & H. Sievert (Eds): 423-429, Cardiotext, Minneapolis, MN, USA

[40] Kramer, P. (2010). The CardioSEAL/STARFlex family of devices for closure of atrial level defects. In: *Transcatheter closure of ASDs and PFOs: A comprehensive assessment*, Z. M. Hijazi, T. Feldman, M. H. Abdullah A Al-Qbandi, & H. Sievert (Eds): 483-399, Cardiotext, Minneapolis, MN, USA

[41] Kretschmar, O.; Sglimbea, A.; Daehnert, I.; et al. (2010). Interventional closure of atrial septal defects with the Solysafe Septal Occluder--preliminary results in children. *Int J Cardiol*, Vol. 143, No. 3, pp. 373-377

[42] Krizanic, F.; Krizanic, F.; Sievert, H.; et al. (2010). The Occlutech Figulla PFO and ASD Occluder: A New Nitinol Wire Mesh Device for Closure of Atrial Septal Defects. *J Invasive Cardiol*, Vol. 22, No. 4, pp. 182–187

[43] Krizanic, F.; Sievert, H.; Pfeiffer, D.; et al.(2008). Clinical evaluation of a novel occluder device (Occlutech) for percutaneous transcatheter closure of patent foramen ovale (PFO). *Clin Res Cardiol*, Vol. 97, No. 12, pp. 872- 877

[44] Krizanic, F.; Sievert, H.; Pfeiffer, D.; et al. (2010).The Occlutech Figulla PFO and ASD occluder: a new nitinol wiremesh device for closure of atrial septal defects. J Invasive Cardiol, Vol. 22, No. 4, pp. 182-187

[45] 45. Lammers, A. E.; Derrick, G.; Haworth, S. G.; et al. (2007). Efficacy and long-term patency of fenestrated Amplatzer devices in children. *Catheter Cardiovasc Interv*, Vol. 70, No. 4, pp. 578-584

[46] Latson, L. A. (1993). Transcatheter closure of atrial septal defects. In: *Transcatheter Therapy in Pediatric Cardiology,* P. S. Rao (ed): 335-348, Wiley-Liss, New York, NY, USA
[47] Latson, L.; Zahn, E. & Wilson N. (2000). HELEX septal occluder for closure of atrial septal defects. *Curr Intervent Cardiol Rep,* Vol. 2, No. 3, pp. 268-273
[48] Lertsapcharoen, P.; Khongphatthanayothin, A.; Srimahachota, S. & Leelanukrom, R. (2008). Self-expanding platinum-coated nitinol devices for transcatheter closure of atrial septal defect: prevention of nickel release. *J Invasive Cardiol,* Vol. 20, No. 6, pp. 279-283
[49] Lewis, F. J. & Tauffic, M. (1953). Closure of atrial septal defects with the aid of hypothermia: experimental accomplishments and the report of one successful case. *Surg,* Vol. 33, No. 1, pp. 52-59
[50] Lloyd, T. R.; Rao, P. S.; Beekman, R. H., III.; et al. (1994). Atrial septal defect occlusion with the buttoned device: a multi-institutional U.S. trial. *Am J Cardiol,* Vol. 73, No. 4, pp. 286-291
[51] Lock, J. E. ; Cockerham J. T.; Keane, J. F.; et al. (1987). Transcatheter umbrella closure of congenital heart defects. *Circulation,* Vol. 75, No. 3, pp. 593-599
[52] Lock, J. E. ; Rome, J. J.; Davis, R.; et al. (1989). Transcatheter closure of atrial septal defects: experimental studies. *Circulation,* Vol. 79, No. 5, pp. 1091-1099
[53] Masura, J.; Gavora, P.; Formanek, A. & Hijazi, Z. M. (1997). Transcatheter closure of secundum atrial septal defects using the new self-centering Amplatzer septal occluder: initial human experience. *Cathet Cardiovasc Diagn,* Vol. 42, No. 4, pp. 388-393
[54] Mills, N. L. & King, T. D. (1976). Nonoperative closure of left-to-right shunts. *J Thorac Cardiovasc Surg, Vol.* 72, No. 3, pp. 371-378
[55] Mullen, M. J.; Hildick-Smith, D.; De Giovanni, J. V.; et al. (2006). BioSTAR Evaluation STudy (BEST): a prospective, multicenter, phase I clinical trial to evaluate the feasibility, efficacy, and safety of the BioSTAR bioabsorbable septal repair implant for the closure of atrial-level shunts. *Circulation,* Vol. 114, No. 18, pp. 1962-1967
[56] Murphy, J. G.; Gersh, B. J.; McGoon, M. D.; et al. (1990). Long-term outcome after surgical repair of isolated atrial septal defect. *New Engl J Med,* Vol. 323, No. 24, pp. 1645-1650
[57] Pastorek, J. S.; Allen, H. D. & Davis, J. T. (1994). Current outcomes of surgical closure of secundum atrial septal defect. *Am J Cardiol,* Vol. 74, No. 2, pp. 175-179
[58] Pavcnik, D.; Takulve, K.; Uchida, B. T.; et al. (2010). Biodisk: a new device for closure of patent foramen ovale: a feasibility study in swine. *Catheter Cardiovasc Interv,* Vol. 75, No. 6, pp. 861-867
[59] Pavcnik, D.; Wright, K. C. & Wallace, S. (1993). Monodisk: device for percutaneous transcatheter closure of cardiac septal defects. *Cardiovasc Intervent Radiol, Vol.* 16, No. 5, pp. 308-312
[60] Pedra, C. A. C.; Pihkala, J.; Lee, K-J.; et al. (2000). Transcatheter closure of the atrial septal defects using the CardioSeal implant. *Heart,* Vol. 84, No. 3, pp. 320-326
[61] Perry, S. B.; Van der Velde, M. E.; Bridges, N. D.; et al. (1993). Transcatheter closure of atrial and ventricular septal defects. *Herz,* Vol. 18, No. 2, pp. 135-142

[62] Prieto, L. R.; Foreman, C. K.; Cheatham, J. P.; et al. (1996). Intermediate-term outcome of transcatheter secundum atrial septal defect closure using Bard clamshell septal umbrella. *Am J Cardiol,* Vol. 78, No. 11, pp. 1310-1312

[63] Rao, P. S. Buttoned Device. (2003) In: *Catheter based devices for the treatment of non-coronary cardiovascular disease in adults and children,* P. S. Rao & M. J. Kern (Eds): 17-34, Lippincott Williams & Wilkins, Philadelphia, PA, USA

[64] Rao, P. S.; Berger, F.; Rey, C.; et al. (2000). Transvenous occlusion of secundum atrial septal defects with 4th generation buttoned device: comparison with 1st, 2nd and 3rd generation devices. *J Am Coll Cardiol, Vol.* 36, No. 2, pp. 583-592

[65] Rao, P. S.; Chander, J. S. & Sideris, E. B. (1997). Role of inverted buttoned device in transcatheter occlusion of atrial septal defects or patent foramen ovale with right-to-left shunting associated with previously operated complex congenital cardiac anomalies. *Am J Cardiol,* Vol. 80, No. 7, pp. 914-921

[66] Rao, P. S. Ende, D. J.; Wilson, A. D.; et al. (1995). Follow-up results of transcatheter occlusion of atrial septal defects with buttoned device. *Cand J Cardiol, Vol.* 11, No. 8, pp. 695-701

[67] Rao, P. S.; Palacios, I. F.; Bach, R. G.; et al. (2001). Platypnea- Orthodeoxia Syndrome: Management by Transcatheter Buttoned Device Implantation. *Cathet Cardiovasc Intervent,* Vol. 54, No. 1, pp. 77-82

[68] Rao, P. S. & Sideris, E. B. (1995). Transcatheter occlusion of cardiac defects [letter].*Br Heart J,* Vol. 73, No. 6, pp. 585-586

[69] Rao, P. S. & Sideris, E. B. (1998). Buttoned device closure of the atrial septal defect. *J Interventional Cardiol, Vol.* 11, No. 5, pp. 467-484

[70] Rao, P. S. & Sideris, E. B. (2001). Centering-on-demand buttoned device: Its role in transcatheter occlusion of atrial septal defects. *J Intervent Cardiol,* Vol. 14, No. 1, pp. 81-89

[71] Rao, P. S.; Sideris, E. B. & Chopra, P. S. (1991). Catheter closure of atrial septal defect: successful use in a 3.6 kg infant. *Am Heart J,* Vol. 121, No. 6, pp. 1826-1829

[72] Rao, P. S.; Sideris, E. B.; Haddad, J.; et al. (1993). Transcatheter occlusion of patent ductus arteriosus with adjustable buttoned device: initial clinical experience. *Circulation,* Vol. 88, No. 3, pp. 1119-1126

[73] Rao, P. S.; Sideris, E. B.; Hausdorf, G.; et al. (1994). International experience with secundum atrial septal defect occlusion by the buttoned device. *Am Heart J,* Vol. 128, No. 5, pp. 1022-1035

[74] Rao, P. S.; Sideris, E. B.; Rey, C.; et al. (1998). Echo-Doppler follow-up evaluation after transcatheter occlusion of atrial septal defects with the buttoned device. In: *Proceedings of the Second World Congress of Pediatric Cardiology and Cardiac Surgery,* Y. Imai & K. Momma (Eds): 197-200, Futura Publishing Co, Armonk, NY, USA

[75] Rao, P. S.; Wilson, A. D.; Levy, J. M.; et al. (1992a). Role of "buttoned" double-disc device in the management of atrial septal defects. *Am Heart J,* Vol. 123, No. 1, pp. 191-200

[76] Rao, P. S, Wilson, A. D.; Chopra, P. S. (1992b). Transcatheter closure of atrial septal defects by "buttoned" devices. *Am J Cardiol,* Vol. 69, No. 12, pp. 1056-1061

[77] Rashkind, W. J. (1975). Experimental transvenous closure of atrial and ventricular septal defects. *Circulation,* Vol. 52, Suppl-II-8

[78] Rashkind, W. J. (1983). Transcatheter treatment of congenital heart disease. *Circulation,* Vol. 67, No. 4, pp. 711-716
[79] Rashkind, W. J. & Cuaso, C. E. (1977). Transcatheter closure of atrial septal defects in children. *Eur J Cardiol,* Vol. 8, No. pp. 119-120
[80] Rashkind, W. J.; Mullins, C. E.; Hellenbrand, W. E.; et al. (1987). Non-surgical closure of patent ductus arteriosus: clinical applications of the Rashkind PDA occluder system. *Circulation,* Vol. 75, No. 3, pp. 583-592
[81] Rashkind, W. J.; Tait, M. A. & Gibson, R. J., Jr. (1985). Interventional cardiac catheterization in congenital heart disease. *Internat J Cardiol,* Vol. 7, No. 1, pp. 1-11
[82] Redington, A. N. & Rigby, M. L. (1994). Transcatheter closure of interatrial communication with a modified umbrella device. *Br Heart J,* Vol. 72, No. 4, pp. 372-377
[83] Rickers, C.; Hamm, C.; Stern, H.; et al. (1998). Percutaneous closure of secundum atrial septal defect with a new self centering device ("angel wings"). *Heart,* Vol. 80, No. 5, pp. 517-521
[84] Rome, J. J.; Keane, J. F.; Perry, S. B.; et al. (1990). Double-umbrella closure of atrial defects: initial clinical applications. *Circulation,* Vol. 82, No. 3, pp. 751-758
[85] Ryan, C.; Opolski, S.; Wright, J.; et al. (1998). Structural considerations in the development of the CardioSeal septal occluder. In: *Proceedings of the Second World Congress of Pediatric Cardiology and Cardiac Surgery,* Y. Imai & K. Momma (Eds): 191-193, Futura Publishing Co, Armonk, NY, USA
[86] Sharafuddin, M. J. A.; Gu, X.; Titus, J. L.; et al. (1997). Transvenous closure of secundum atrial septal defects: preliminary results with a new self-expanding Nitinol prosthesis in a swine model. *Circulation,* Vol. 95, No. 8, pp. 2162-2168
[87] Schneider, M.; Babic, U.; Thomsen, B. A.; et al., (1995). Das ASDOS-Implantat: Tierexperimentelle Erprobung. *Z Kardiologie,* Vol. 84: (Suppl.) pp. 751
[88] Schraeder, R.; Fassbender, D. & Strasser, R. H. (2003). PFO-star for closure of patent foramen ovale in patients with presumed paradoxical embolism. In: *Catheter based devices for the treatment of non-coronary cardiovascular disease in adults and children,* P. S. Rao & M. J Kern (Eds): 103-109, Lippincott Williams & Wilkins, Philadelphia, PA, USA
[89] Sideris, E. B. (2003). Wireless devices. In: *Catheter based devices for the treatment of non-coronary cardiovascular disease in adults and children,* P. S. Rao, & M. J Kern (Eds): 79-84, Lippincott Williams & Wilkins, Philadelphia, PA, USA
[90] Sideris, E. B.; Chiang, C. W.; Zhang, J. C. & Wang, W. S. (1999a). Transcatheter correction of heart defects by detachable balloon buttoned devices: A feasibility study. *J Am Coll Cardiol,* Vol. 33 No. 2, Suppl A, p. 528
[91] Sideris, B. E.; Coulson, J. D. & Sideris, E. B. (2010). Transcatheter patch device. In: *Transcatheter closure of ASDs and PFOs: A comprehensive assessment,* Z. M. Hijazi, T. Feldman, M. H. Abdullah A Al-Qbandi, & H. Sievert (Eds): 373-384, Cardiotext, Minneapolis, MN, USA
[92] Sideris, E.; Kaneva, A.; Sideris, S. & Moulopoulos, S. (2000a). Transcatheter atrial septal defect occlusion in piglets by balloon detachable devices. *Catheter Cardiovasc Interventions,* Vol. 51, No. 4, pp. 529-534

[93] Sideris, E. B.; Leung, M.; Yoon, J. H.; et al. (1996). Occlusion of large atrial septal defects with a centering device: early clinical experience. *Am Heart J*, Vol. 131, No. 2, pp. 356-359

[94] Sideris, E. B.; Sideris, S. E.; Fowlkes, J. P.; et al. (1990a). Transvenous atrial septal occlusion in piglets using a "buttoned" double-disc device. *Circulation*, Vol. 81, No. 1, pp. 312-318

[95] Sideris, E. B.; Sideris, E. E.; Kaneva, A.; et al. (1999b). Transcatheter occlusion of experimental atrial septal defects by wireless occluders and patches (abstract). *Cardiol Young*, Vol. 9, Suppl, p. 92

[96] Sideris, E. B.; Sideris, S. E.; Thanopoulos, B. D.; et al. (1990b). Transvenous atrial septal defect occlusion by the "buttoned" device. *Am J Cardiol*, Vol. 66, No. 20, pp. 1524-1526

[97] Sideris, E. B.; Rey, C.; Schrader, R.; et al. (1997). Occlusion of large atrial septal defects by buttoned devices; comparison of centering and the fourth generation devices [abstract]. *Circulation*, Vol. 96, No. 8S, p. I-99

[98] Sideris, E.; Toumanides, S.; Alekyan, B.; et al. (2000b). Transcatheter patch correction of atrial septal defects: Experimental validation and early clinical experience. *Circulation*, Vol. 102: (Suppl) II, p. 588

[99] Sievert, H.; Babic, U. U.; Ensslen, R.; et al. (1995). Transcatheter closure of large atrial septal defects with the Babic system. *Cathet Cardiovasc Diagn*, Vol. 36: No. 3, pp. 232-240

[100] Sievert, H.; Babic, U. U.; Hausdorf, G.; et al. (1998). Transcatheter closure of atrial septal defect and patent foramen ovale with ASDOS device, a multi-institutional European trial. *Am J Cardiol*, Vol. 82, No. 11, pp. 1405-1413

[101] Stolt, V. S.; Chessa, M.; Aubry, P.; et al. (2010). Closure of ostium secundum atrial septum defect with the Atriasept occluder: early European experience. *Catheter Cardiovasc Interv*, Vol. 75, No. 7, pp. 1091-1095

[102] Thomsen-Bloch, A. (1995).Closure of Atrial Septal Defects with Catheter Technique: An animal experimental study. Diploma Thesis, Aarhus University Hospital, Denmark

[103] Turner, D. R. & Forbes, T. J. (2010). Cardia devices. In: *Transcatheter closure of ASDs and PFOs: A comprehensive assessment*, Z. M. Hijazi, T. Feldman, M. H. Abdullah A Al-Qbandi, & H. Sievert (Eds): 407-416, Cardiotext, Minneapolis, MN, USA

[104] Worms, A. M.; Rey, C.; Bourlan, F.; et al. (1996). French experience in the closure of atrial septal defects of the ostium secundum type with Sideris buttoned occluder. *Arch Mal Coeur Vaiss*, Vol. 89, No. 5, pp. 509-515

[105] Zahn, E.; Cheatham, J.; Latson, L. & Wilson, N. (1999). Results of in vivo testing of a new Nitinol ePTTEF septal occlusion device. *Cathet Cardiovasc Intervent*, Vol. 47, No. 1, pp. 124

[106] Zahn, E.; Wilson, N.; Cutright, W. & Latson, L. (2001). Development and testing of the HELEX septal occluder, a new expanded polytetraflouroethylene atrial septal defect occlusion system. *Circulation*, Vol. 104, No. 6, pp. 711-716

[107] Zamora, R.; Rao ,P. S.; Lloyd, T.R.; et al. (1998). Intermediate-term results of Phase I FDA trials of buttoned device occlusion of secundum atrial septal defects. *J Am Coll Cardiol*, Vol. 31, No. 3, pp. 674-678

[108] Zamora, R.; Rao, P. S. & Sideris, E. B. (2000). Buttoned device for atrial septal defect occlusion. *Current Intervent Cardiol Reports,* Vol. 2, No. 2, pp. 167-176

6

Role of Transesophageal Echocardiography in Transcatheter Occlusion of Atrial Septal Defects

Gurur Biliciler-Denktas
University of Texas Health Science Center Houston, Division of Pediatric Cardiology
USA

1. Introduction

The incidence of atrial septal defect (ASD) is 1 in 1000 live births and account up to one third of the acyanotic shunts in the adult population. (Brickner et al. 2000; Yared et al. 2009) Patent foramen ovale (PFO) is found more than 25% of the adults. (Yared, Baggish et al. 2009) Historically, surgical closure of ASDs has been the most common therapy until new catheter-based techniques began to develop pioneered by King and Mills in 1975. (King et al. 1976; Yared et al. 2009) Currently, transcatheter closure of ASDs and PFOs is preferred to surgery in otherwise uncomplicated and favorable anatomy cases because it is technically simple and is associated with negligible morbidity and mortality. These procedures are performed for hemodynamically significant left to right shunting, to prevent stroke from recurrent paradoxical embolism and for the platypnea orthodeoxia syndrome. In addition to the above, closure of the surgically created fenestrations after Fontan operations and also baffle leaks after Mustard and Senning surgeries are all performed in the catheterization laboratory. (Hanrath 2001; Sengupta & Khandheria 2005) Several echocardiographic techniques including transthoracic echocardiography (TTE), transesophageal echocardiography (TEE), intracardiac echocardiography (ICE) and real time three-dimensional transesophageal echocardiography (3D TEE) are being used by many centers. (Silvestry et al. 2009) In this chapter, we will review the role of TEE in transcatheter occlusion of atrial septal defects.

2. Development of interatrial septum

A good knowledge of the cardiac anatomy is needed for the echocardiographers to identify the structures and share them in a common language with the rest of the team involved in the care of the patient before, during and after the procedure.

The major septa of the heart are formed between the 27th and 37th days of development. One method by which a septum may be formed involves actively growing masses of tissue that approach each other until they fuse dividing the lumen into two separate canals (symmetrical growth). Septum may also be formed by active growth of a single tissue mass that continues to expand until it reaches the opposite side of the lumen (asymmetrical growth). (Fig. 1)

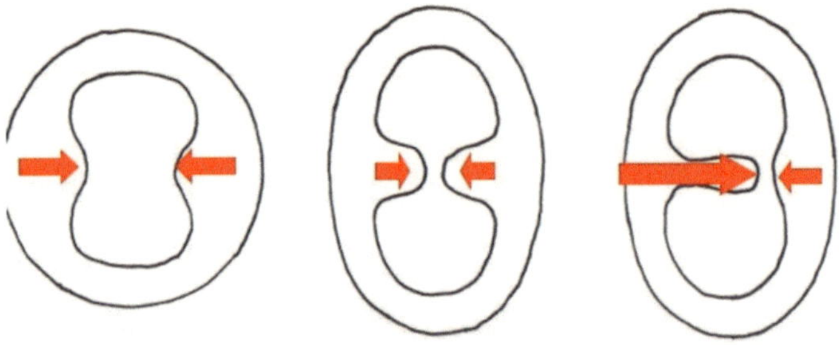

Fig. 1. Formation of septa. Symmetrical (middle) and asymmetrical (right) growth (Courtesy of Dr. Stephen W. Carmichael)

Atrium starts as a common chamber. At the end of the 4th week, a sickle cell shaped crest grows from the roof of the common atrium into the lumen. This is the first portion of the septum primum.

The opening between the lower rim of the septum primum and the endocardial cushions is the ostium primum. (Fig. 2)

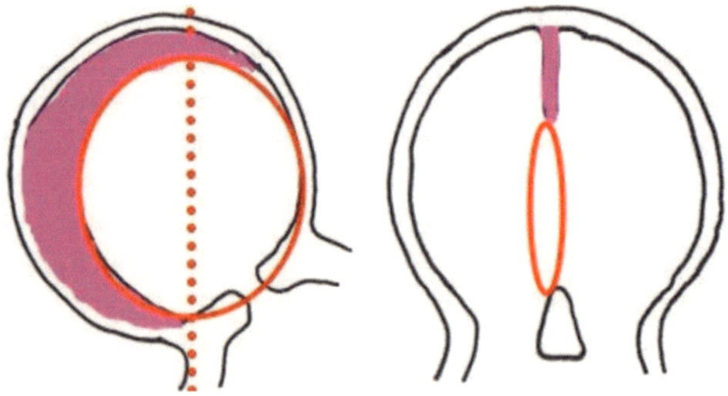

Fig. 2. Septum primum (in pink) and ostium primum (in red) (Courtesy of Dr. Stephen W. Carmichael)

With further development, extensions of the endocardial cushions grow along the edge of the septum primum closing the ostium primum. Before closure is complete, cell death produces perforations in the upper portions of the septum. (Fig. 3)

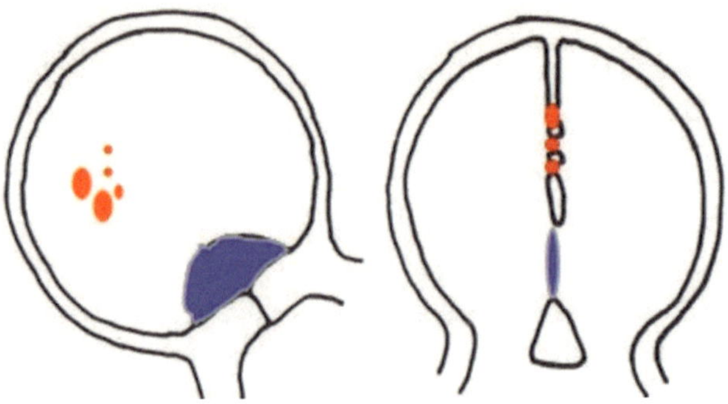

Fig. 3. Closure of ostium primum (in blue) and perforations in the septum (in red) (Courtesy of Dr. Stephen W. Carmichael)

Holes in septum primum coalesce to form ostium secundum. When the lumen of the right atrium expands as a result of the incorporation of the sinus horn, a new crescent shaped fold appears. Septum secundum begins to grow over ostium secundum. Septum secundum is to the right of septum primum and is more rigid. (Fig. 4)

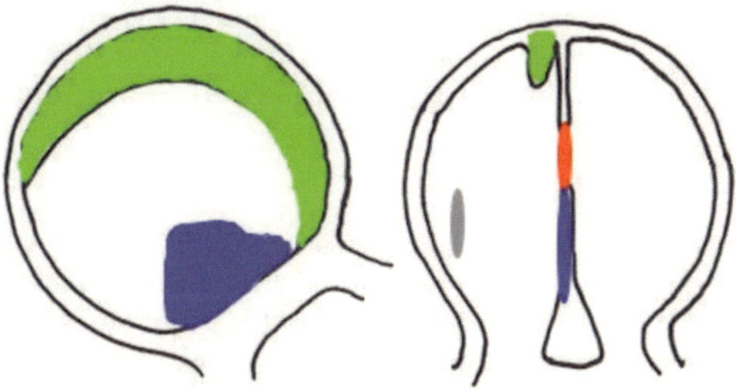

Fig. 4. Septum secundum (in green), septum primum (in blue) and ostium secundum (in red) (Courtesy of Dr. Stephen W. Carmichael)

Free concave edge of the septum secundum begins to overlap the ostium secundum. The tunnel like opening left by the septum secundum is the foramen ovale. Eventually within the first few years of life, the septum secundum fuses with the septum primum in most of the population thus separating the two atria. (Fig. 5)

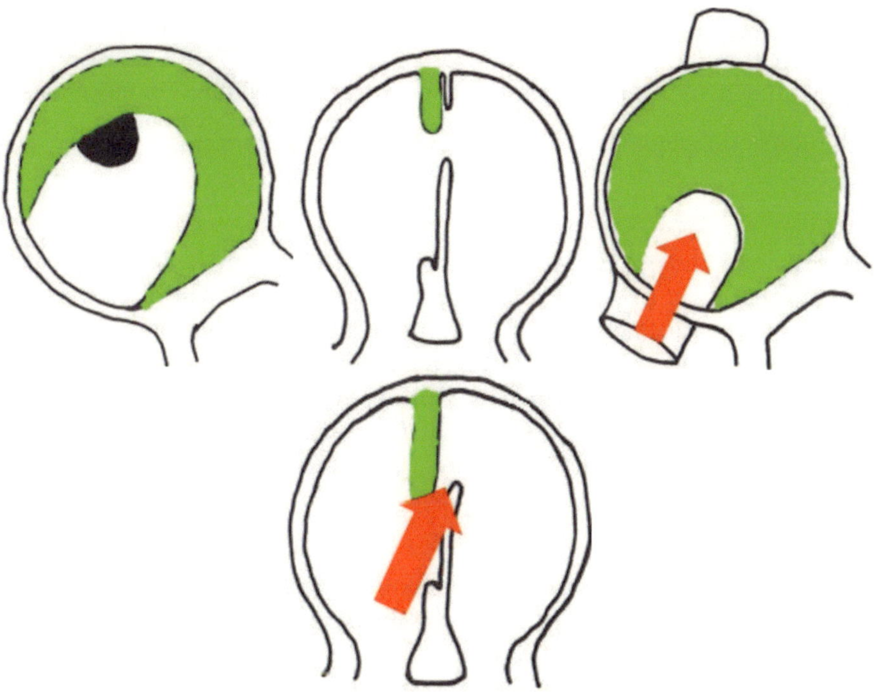

Fig. 5. Septum secundum (in green) and foramen ovale (in red arrow) (Courtesy of Dr. Stephen W. Carmichael)

Ostium secundum ASDs are caused either by excessive cell death and resorption of the septum primum or by inadequate development of the septum secundum.

PFO which is the result of lack of fusion between the septum primum and the septum secundum is not considered a true ASD and stays functionally closed as long as the left atrial pressure is higher than the right atrial pressure. There is a potential for right to left shunting resulting in paradoxical embolism and stroke if the right atrial pressure rises (mostly observed with valsalva) enough to open the PFO. (Johri et al. 2011)

3. Echocardiographic techniques

Echocardiography has been the widely used imaging technique that complements the fluoroscopy during closure of ASDs and PFOs. Compared to computed tomography and magnetic resonance imaging, echocardiography has the major advantage of being portable and real time. In this way, echocardiography can be performed before, during and after transcatheter interventions. (Silvestry et al. 2009) Even though fluoroscopy is the main imaging modality during interventional procedures, it does not provide direct assessment of cardiac anatomy as good as echocardiography. In addition to defining the intracardiac structures important in the ASD closure process, echocardiography is helpful in showing the relationship between catheters or devices and the adjacent structures. (Brochet & Vahanian 2010) The use of echocardiography as an adjunct to fluoroscopy has decreased the amount of total fluoro time to close an ASD.

Once the diagnosis of ASD or PFO and a decision to close it has been made, atrial septum should be assessed immediately before the procedure in the cardiac catheterization laboratory to confirm the diagnosis, during the procedure to help with device occlusion and after the procedure to reconfirm the success of the procedure without complications.

There are multiple techniques for the imaging of the atrial septum.

3.1 TTE

TTE is the simplest technique to use. It can show the device in multiple planes but does not have adequate imaging of the lower rim of the atrial septal tissue, which is above the inferior vena cava (IVC) especially after device placement. In addition to this, since the distance from the septum to the transducer is farther in TTE than TEE or ICE, the color imaging at the atrial septal level may be suboptimal. Access to the patient's body through the sterile field also poses a problem. Even though TTE may be the initial diagnostic tool, it is infrequently used in the catheterization laboratory to aid in ASD closures. (Silvestry et al. 2009)

3.2 TEE

In contrast to TTE, TEE offers better image resolution and definition of anatomy during the transcatheter closure of ASDs. It has become the standard imaging modality in many centers to monitor and guide interventional procedures because of its easy application, lower cost, portability and real time imaging. It is mostly agreed that TEE is superior to fluoroscopy in defining the defect margins and to position the device and/or its arms. (Hanrath 2001) The main limitation of TEE is the need for general anesthesia. (Brochet & Vahanian 2010) It also requires a dedicated echocardiographer to perform the study. TEE in ASD closure will be discussed further in the rest of the chapter.

3.3 ICE

ICE has been introduced to cardiac imaging techniques more than 10 years ago. It has evolved from cross sectional imaging using a rotating transducer to sector based imaging using a phased-array transducer. There are three ICE catheters available with respective ultrasound systems. Most frequently used ones are 8F or 10 F ultrasound catheters. Some centers prefer ICE to other imaging modalities because of its superiority in imaging especially the inferior rim of the atrial septum, which is important in decision making to close the defect. (Kim et al. 2009) It is advantageous to TEE mostly because it avoids the need for general anesthesia. The cost of the catheter is one of the main drawbacks of using ICE. Even though closure of PFO under the guidance of ICE is safe and effective, ICE may not be sensitive enough to detect all patients with right to left shunting. (Van et al. 2010; Pedra, Fleishman et al. 2011) In addition to this, limited field view for far field device complications, the need for a second venous sheath, the requirement for additional training, potential trigger of atrial arrhythmias are among the disadvantages of ICE. In the setting of a single operator, it may be a more challenge to manipulate the ICE catheter at the same time the closure device. It is up to the center and the interventionalist to prefer ICE to other imaging techniques and there are many catheterization laboratories and interventionalists who prefer this technique during transcatheter closure of ASDs. (Kim et al. 2009; Yared et al. 2009)

3.4 3D TEE

After the introduction of 3D TTE during interventions, a more practical technique, 3D TEE was developed. Real time 3D TEE images have high spatial and temporal resolution that allows detailed views of the cardiac structures. (Lee et al. 2010; Tsang et al. 2011) The use of 3D TEE acquired en face views of the defect and surrounding structures allows accurate measurement of the ASD and any other additional defects like fenestrations. Since the same probe can be used for 2D TEE and 3D TEE imaging and the operator can switch in between the two modalities, this method has become one of the newer and promising techniques in evaluation of the atrial septum during ASD device occlusion.

4. ASD/PFO closure devices

Currently there are a number of devices approved in the USA for closure of ASDs and some of these are also used off label for closure of PFOs. It is very important for the echocardiographer to be familiar with these devices, their design and release mechanisms since the method of implantation is different and unique for each device. (Silvestry et al. 2009)

Atrial septal defect occlusion devices are categorized into two as non-self centered or single pin device and the waist or self-centered device. The cribriform device- AGA Amplatzer multi fenestrated septal occluder (AGA, Plymouth. Minnesota USA) (Fig. 6) and the Gore Helex septal occluder (GL Gore & Associates, Flagstaff, Arizona, USA) (Fig. 7) are among the family of single pin devices. Both the Cribriform and the Gore Helex devices are approved for closure of small ASDs but are widely used for PFO closure as off label indication. The self-centered devices have two atrial disks that connect with a waist. AGA Amplatzer septal occluder (AGA) (Fig. 6) and the NMT CardioSeal StarFlex septal occluder (NMT Medical, Boston, Massachusetts, USA) (Fig. 7) are the two self centered devices available for closure of ASDs in the USA.

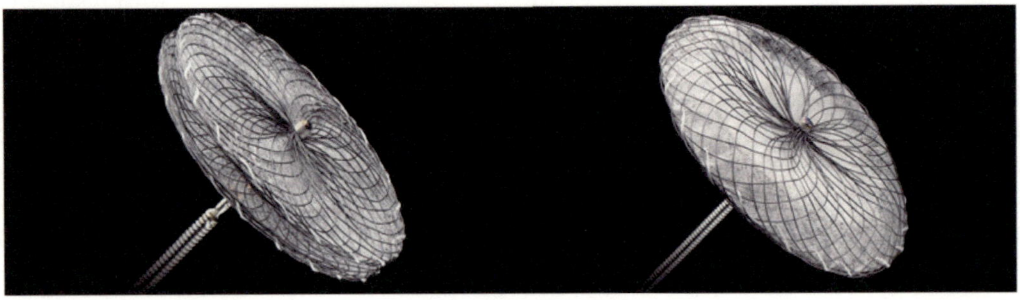

Fig. 6. AGA Amplatzer. Multi Fenestrated Septal Occluder (left) and Septal Occluder (right)

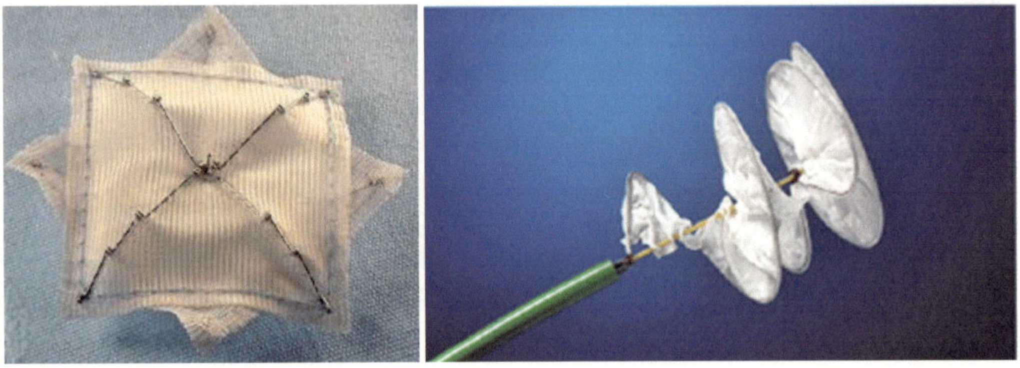

Fig. 7. CardioSeal StarFlex Septal Occluder (left) and Gore Helex Septal Occluder (right)

5. TEE in ASD device closure

5.1 TEE protocol

Even though ASD/PFO closure evaluation asks for certain measurements, for all cases, it is very important to follow a protocol using multiplane views and available windows from gastric to mid and upper esophagus to complete a segmental approach used in evaluation of congenital heart disease. (Fig. 8) In this way, the previous findings seen by other echocardiography modalities will be confirmed and any additional defects will not be missed. (Masani 2001) Many centers already are using TEE protocols that they have developed and these can be incorporated into TEE in interventional studies.

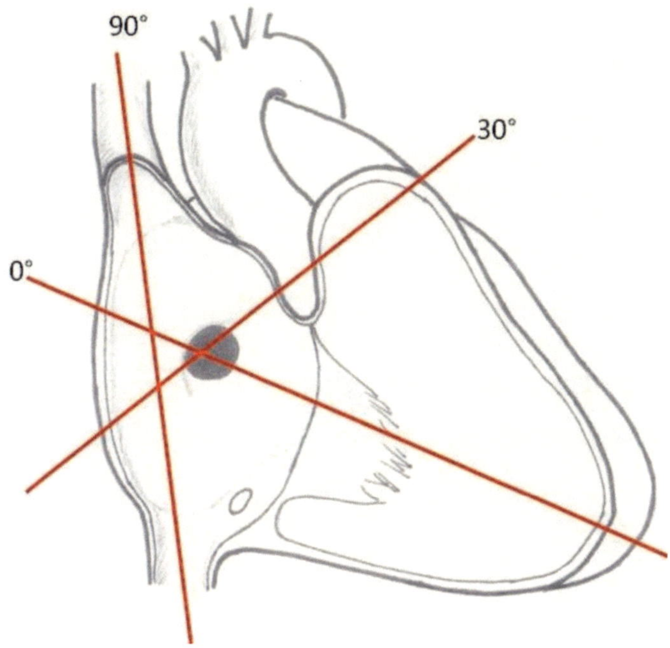

Fig. 8. Multiplane views of the atrial septum. (Courtesy of Dr. Duraisamy Balaguru)

5.2 Imaging of atrial septum pre-, during and post-, device closure

The goals of TEE are: detailed imaging of the defect and its relation to the surrounding structures, identification of patients with suitable anatomy for device closure of their ASD/PFO and guidance for the device positioning and deployment. (Brochet & Vahanian 2010) It should also be kept in mind that the rotation of the transducer to specific angles is a good initial guide but not a strict rule. The defects and other normal structures of the heart may be imaged at closer but different angles.

5.2.1 Pre-procedure

1. Evaluation of the entire atrial septum and its surrounding structures; exclusion of additional defects that may render the defect unsuitable for closure
2. Defining the defect: ASD vs. PFO
3. Color Doppler imaging of the defect and definition of the shunt (left to right, right to left) at rest, with Valsalva
4. In cases of PFO requiring further information of the shunt, injection of agitated saline micro bubbles at rest and with Valsalva to visualize any right to left shunting
5. Measurement of the defect number and size
6. Maximal dimensions of the length of the atrial septum and distance of the ASD from the surrounding structures (rims) (Fig. 12)
7. Measurement of the diameter of the stretched balloon across the defect when a sizing balloon is used and identification of any residual left to right shunting (Fig. 15)

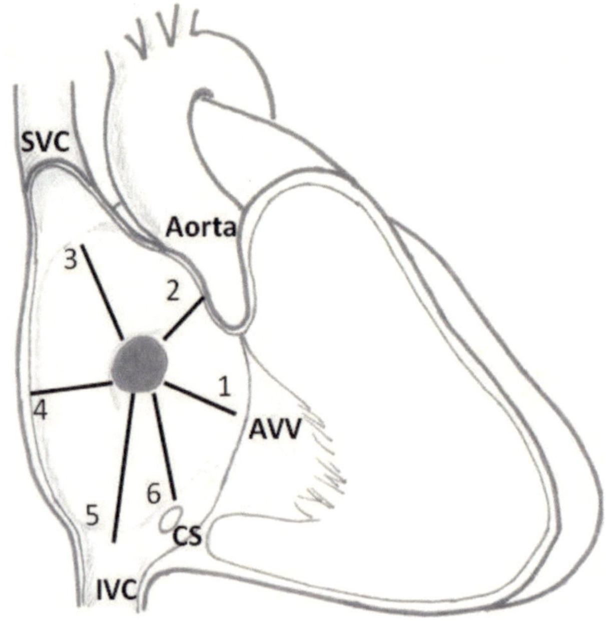

Fig. 9. Secundum atrial septal defect with surrounding rims. (1. Atrioventricular valve rim; 2. Aortic rim; 3. SVC rim; 4. Posterior rim; 5. IVC rim; 6. Coronary sinus rim) (Courtesy of Dr. Duraisamy Balaguru)

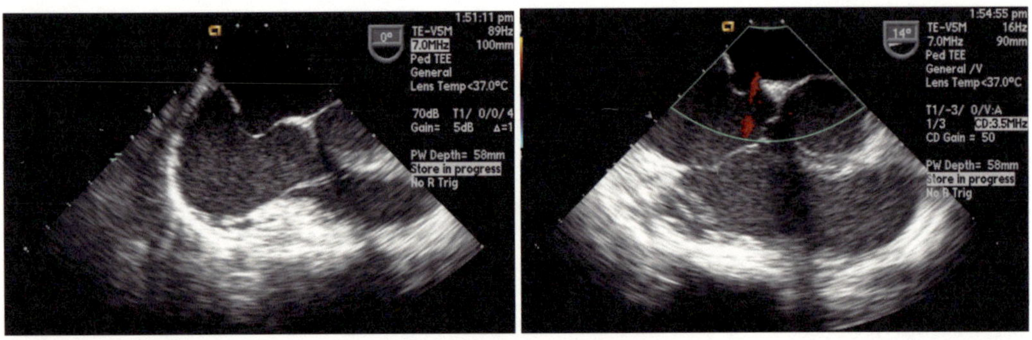

Fig. 10. Atrial septal aneurysm with small left to right shunting

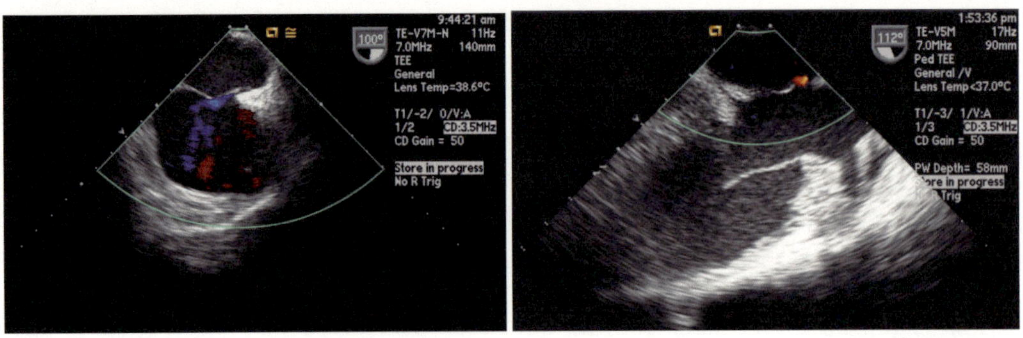

Fig. 11. PFO with bidirectional shunting.

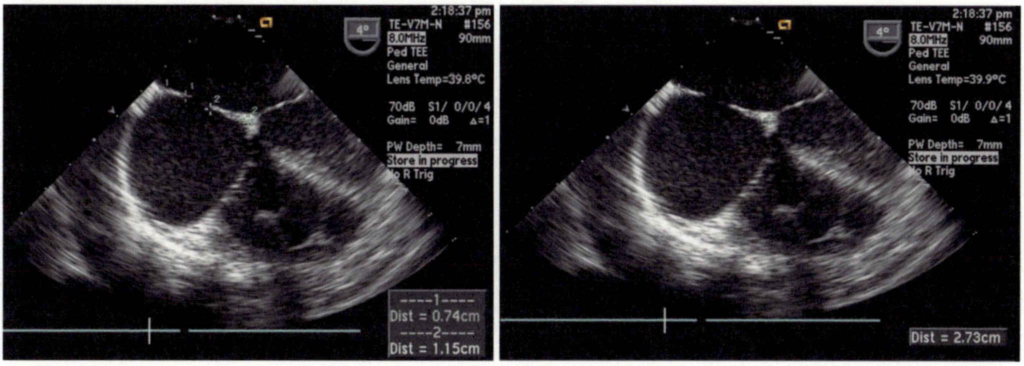

Fig. 12. Four chamber view. Septal defect size, rims (left) and total atrial septal length (right) measurements

A PFO is defined as any anatomical communication through the foramen ovale and a stretched PFO is defined as any left to right flow on color Doppler imaging seen at rest or intermittently. Furthermore, an atrial septal aneurysm is defined as 11-15 mm of total movement of a 15 mm base of atrial tissue. (Silvestry et al. 2009) Sinus venosus, ostium primum or coronary sinus defects cannot be closed by transcatheter intervention and require surgical closure. In addition to this, associated abnormalities of the superior and inferior vena cava, coronary sinus, pulmonary veins and atrioventricular valves that may hinder the device closure should be carefully evaluated. Once the defect is diagnosed as a secundum ASD or a PFO, then the number (more than one defect at the atrial septum or fenestrations) and size of the defect needs to be identified. Currently, defects up to 40 mm in diameter and also multiple defects can be successfully closed with percutaneous transcatheter occlusion. (Silvestry et al. 2009) In addition to the size of the defect, the distance of the defect from the surrounding structures called "rims" play an important role in deciding whether a defect can be closed or not. A surrounding rim of 4-5 mm is considered to be adequate for closure except for the aortic rim which could be less. Posterior, superior (SVC) and especially the inferior (IVC) rim are to be investigated and measured from multiple TEE views for accuracy. (Fig. 14) In the cardiac catheterization laboratory, the operators should be very much familiar with the terminology when rims are mentioned. Alternatively, an easier and according to their relation to less complicated definition of the rims may be specific structures. In smaller patients, especially the pediatric population, the total septal length is also crucial since this may limit the size of the device that can be placed successfully without early or late morbidity. (Momenah et al. 2000)

While interrogating the atrial septum, certain views are recommended for measurements. The diameter of the defect and the color Doppler across it should be obtained from midesophageal four chamber, from short axis at the base of the heart, from gastro esophageal junction and from bicaval view and the largest diameter should be considered while deciding on the size of the device. (Fig 12 and 13) Inferior rim of the defect to mitral valve and tricuspid valve and the total septal length can easily be visualized from mid esophageal four chamber view. (Fig. 12) The short axis view at the base of the heart gives the antero-superior rim (to aortic root), posterior rim (to pulmonary vein) and the total septal length. (Fig 13) With the gastro esophageal junction (0°) or oblique (130°) imaging inferior rim of the defect to the coronary sinus can be seen. Bicaval view is the choice for

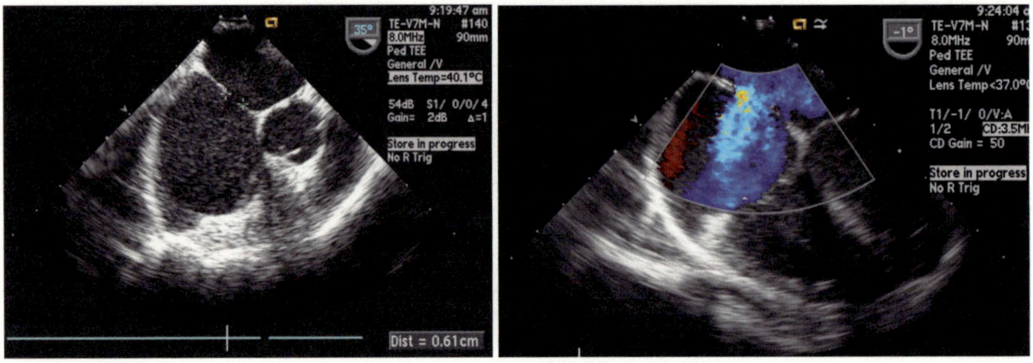

Fig. 13. ASD and aortic rim visualized from short axis view (35°) (left); left to right color flow at ASD (right)

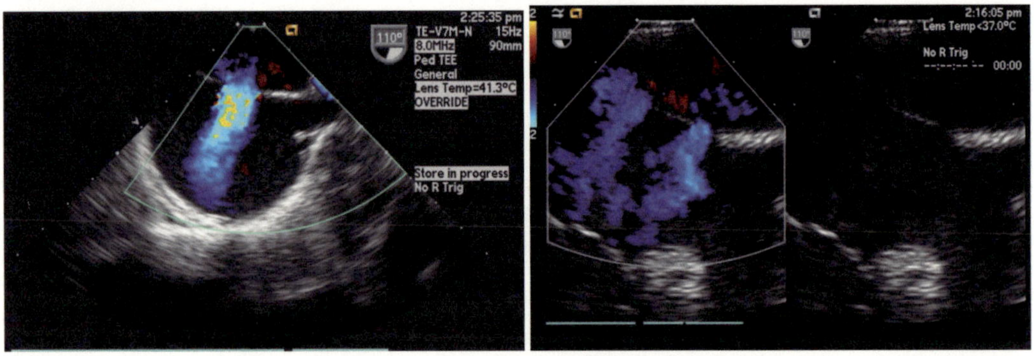

Fig. 14. Bicaval view showing IVC and SVC rims, ASD (left) and fenestrated ASD (right) with left to right shunting

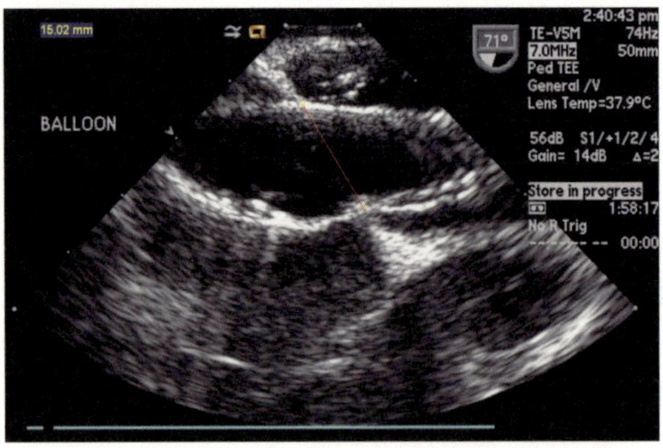

Fig. 15. Balloon sizing of ASD. Note the measurement (in red) at the waist of the stretched balloon

visualization and measurement of the superior rim to superior vena cava and inferior rim to inferior vena cava in addition to the total septal length. (Fig. 14) The color flow entering the RA from vena cava and coronary sinus should not be misdiagnosed. (Masani 2001) Another very important structure is the crista terminalis that extends as a linear structure from the

RA wall close to the IVC to the septum adjacent to the SVC. This structure and the valve of the IVC, Eustachian valve or Chiari network, can both be mistaken as the atrial septum thus ending in a wrong diagnosis. (Masani 2001)

5.2.2 During device closure/deployment

The echocardiographer and the interventionalist work as a team to decide on the device size to be used for ASD/PFO closure. The measurements from both the TEE and cardiac catheterization should be used in choosing the right size device. Once the device is being introduced into the heart and through the defect, the echocardiographer guides the catheterization team with the correct positioning taking into fact the adjacent structures especially AV valves and the entrapment of rims in between the discs (for AGA and Gore Helex septal occluders) and the double umbrella (for NMT CardioSeal). (Fig. 16) Once appropriate placement is confirmed with 2D and no significant left to right shunting seen by color Doppler, the device can then be deployed. (Fig. 17) Small central shunting is frequently seen through the device especially the AGA septal occluders, and this should not hinder the deployment. (Fig. 16) The slight pull of the device by the delivery system is relieved once it is deployed and the device is seen saddling in a much better fashion over the defect.

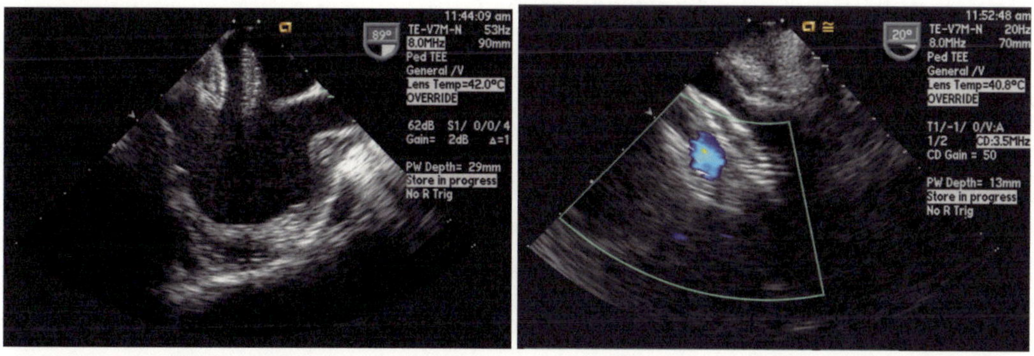

Fig. 16. AGA septal occluder. Note the device malpositioning- vertical to the atrial septum and the ASD rather than parallel (left) and normal central shunting (right)

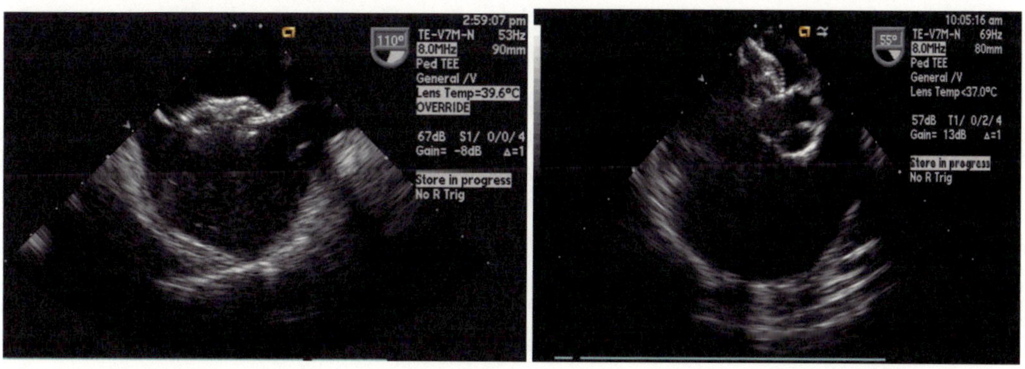

Fig. 17. AGA septal occluder. Correct positioning at bicaval (SVC-IVC) view (left). Straddling the aortic rim (right)

5.2.3 Post device closure

Following deployment, a detailed post procedure TEE should be performed to visualize any impingement on valves, veins and the outflow tract in addition to any residual peripheral shunting. (Fig. 18) In case of acute complications, most of the ASD/PFO occlusion devices can be retrieved in the catheterization laboratory so early post procedure identification of these findings is very important. (Johri et al. 2011)

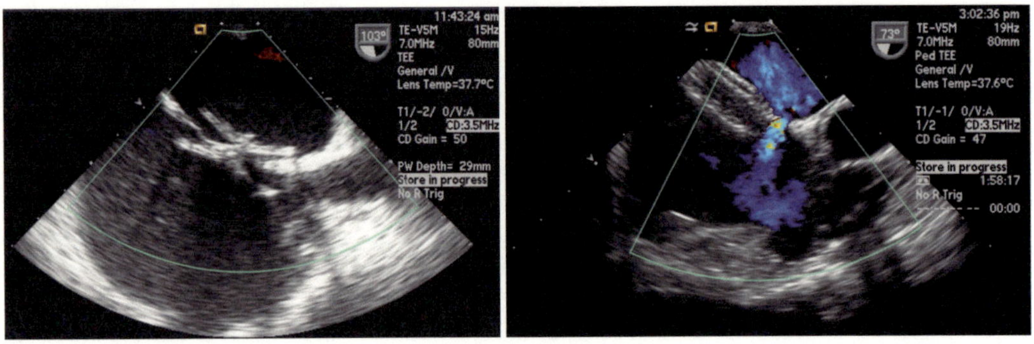

Fig. 18. Gore Helex septal occluder after successful ASD closure (left) and AGA septal occluder with residual peripheral shunting (right)

6. Complications after ASD/PFO device closure

Potential complications after percutaneous device closure of ASDs and PFOs can be categorized into acute/early and chronic/late. In both the acute and late complications TEE plays a very important role. Initially, TEE is helpful in identifying the early complications some of which will be evident in the catheterization laboratory right after deployment.

One of the major but rare complications is device embolization which can embolize to any cardiac chamber or vessel and/or cause valvular dysfunction. Device embolization is commonly secondary to underestimation of the septal defect or the deficiency of the inferior or the superior rims. TEE may be limited in visualization if the device embolizes outside the heart especially beyond the abdominal aorta at the hepatic level or into the peripheral vasculature. (Yared et al. 2009) Once the diagnosis is made by TEE and fluoroscopy, retrieval is attempted in the catheterization laboratory. If unsuccessful, surgical retrieval is done.

Pericardial tamponade though rare is an important complication that may be seen during or acutely after device deployment. Tamponade most frequently is a result of left atrial appendage perforation during the anchoring of the trans septal guide wire though other less commonly encountered reasons may also be from right atrium, right ventricle, or right or left pulmonary vein perforation and though usually a late complication, device erosion through adjacent cardiac tissue. (Yared et al. 2009)

Transient heart block should raise the suspicion of the ASD closure device's impingement on the atrioventricular node. This finding needs to be closely followed afterwards.

Residual shunting seen immediately after device closure may decrease or disappear as the devices endothelizes within several months after deployment. As long as, the residual shunting is not hemodynamically significant, by many, this finding is not considered to be a complication. (Yared et al. 2009)

7. Pitfalls

Even though TEE is one of the most widely used echocardiographic modalities, it also has pitfalls. It requires expert imaging personal to avoid any wrong diagnosis from misinterpretation of normal and abnormal anatomy of the heart, atrial septum and the defect. Even though it is superior to TTE in imaging because the probe in the esophagus is close to the heart, there may still be disturbance in image quality secondary to air within the esophagus and stomach or the air filled trachea or bronchi. In addition, during prolonged monitoring the transducer may reach its heat limit and may need to be turned off until it reaches a cooler temperature. (Sengupta & Khandheria 2005)

8. Conclusion and future directions

During percutaneous closure of ASDs and PFOs, in addition to fluoroscopy, echocardiographic input is of utmost value to the interventionalist. Among the other imaging modalities which include TTE, ICE and 3D TEE, TEE has long been the standard imaging modality in many centers to monitor and guide interventional procedures because of its easy application, lower cost, portability and real time imaging. With the introduction of smaller transducers, it is also used in the smaller patients, especially the pediatric population. It is the preference, comfort and the expertise of the interventionalist and the echocardiographer to choose the best imaging technique for percutaneous ASD/PFO closure. Since TEE has been used for a long time with good results, it still is the choice of imaging in many of the catheterization laboratories; ICE and 3D TEE are the upcoming competitors.

9. References

Brickner, M. E., L. D. Hillis, R. A. Lange (2000). "Congenital heart disease in adults. First of two parts." *N Engl J Med* 342(4): 256-63.

Brochet, E. and A. Vahanian (2010). "Echocardiography in the catheterisation laboratory." *Heart* 96(17): 1409-17.

Hanrath, P. (2001). "Imaging techniques: Transoesophageal Echo-Doppler in cardiology." *Heart* 86(5): 586-92.

Johri, A. M., C. A. Rojas, A. El-Sherif et al. (2011). "Imaging of atrial septal defects: echocardiography and CT correlation." *Heart* 97(17): 1441-53.

Kim, S. S., Z. M. Hijazi, R. M. Lang et al. (2009). "The use of intracardiac echocardiography and other intracardiac imaging tools to guide noncoronary cardiac interventions." *J Am Coll Cardiol* 53(23): 2117-28.

King, T. D., S. L. Thompson, C. Steiner et al. (1976). "Secundum atrial septal defect. Nonoperative closure during cardiac catheterization." *Jama* 235(23): 2506-9.

Lee, A. P., Y. Y. Lam, G. W. K. Yip et al. (2010). "Role of real time three-dimensional transesophageal echocardiography in guidance of interventional procedures in cardiology." *Heart* 96(18): 1485-93.

Masani, N. D. (2001). "Transoesophageal echocardiography in adult congenital heart disease." *Heart* 86 Suppl 2: II30-II40.

Momenah, T. S., D. B. McElhinney, M. M. Brook et al. (2000). "Transesophageal echocardiographic predictors for successful transcatheter closure of defects within the oval fossa using the CardioSEAL septal occlusion device." *Cardiol Young* 10(5): 510-8.

Pedra, C. A., C. Fleishman, S. F. Pedra et al. (2011). "New imaging modalities in the catheterization laboratory." *Curr Opin Cardiol* 26(2): 86-93.

Sengupta, P. P. and B. K. Khandheria (2005). "Transoesophageal echocardiography." *Heart* 91(4): 541-7.

Silvestry, F. E., R. E. Kerber, M. M. Brook et al. (2009). "Echocardiography-guided interventions." *J Am Soc Echocardiogr* 22(3): 213-31; quiz 316-7.

Tsang, W., R. M. Lang, I. Kronzon (2011). "Role of real-time three dimensional echocardiography in cardiovascular interventions." *Heart* 97(10): 850-7.

Van, H., P. Poommipanit, M. Shalaby et al. (2010). "Sensitivity of transcranial Doppler versus intracardiac echocardiography in the detection of right-to-left shunt." *JACC Cardiovasc Imaging* 3(4): 343-8.

Yared, K., A. L. Baggish, J. Solis et al. (2009). "Echocardiographic assessment of percutaneous patent foramen ovale and atrial septal defect closure complications." *Circ Cardiovasc Imaging* 2(2): 141-9.

7

Role of Intracardiac Echocardiography (ICE) in Transcatheter Occlusion of Atrial Septal Defects

Ismael Gonzalez, Qi-Ling Cao and Ziyad M. Hijazi*
Rush Center for Congenital & Structural Heart Disease,
Rush University Medical Center, Chicago, IL,
USA

1. Introduction

Nowadays transcatheter closure of atrial septal defects (ASDs) is a reality in the vast majority of countries; this procedure can be done safely and effectively in skilled hands and with the appropriate devices. Accurate and precise knowledge of the anatomy of the secundum atrial septal defect and the nearby structures is essential for the effectiveness and safe performance of ASD closure. Improvements in ultrasound technology over the last several decades have been particularly useful for guidance during this particular invasive procedure.

Transesophageal echocardiography (TEE) has been the conventional imaging method for guidance in transcatheter closure of ASDs in children and adults; TEE has been shown to be safe and effective for closure of ASDs but in the majority of cases it has to be done under general anesthesia with subsequent increase in the procedure time, increased risks of anesthesia and patient discomfort after the procedure.

Intracardiac echocardiogram (ICE) was developed to provide accurate and precise knowledge of the anatomy of the intracardiac structures. ICE was first used in 1980s for the visualization of the coronary arteries and then it was also used as a guiding tool during radiofrequency ablation and to assist transeptal puncture techniques in difficult cases. It was our group who reported for the first time in 2001 on the use of ICE to guide device closure of ASDs and patent foramen ovale.

Since then, multiple improvements in the ICE catheter have been developed and now it is well recognized imaging tool for guidance of several interventional cardiac and electrophysiological procedures.

Unlike TEE, ICE doesn't require general anesthesia, it provides accurate real time images and the procedure can be done faster with successful results.

2. History

During the 1950s and 1960s, the first ultrasound tipped catheters were introduced because of the advancement in percutaneous procedures in the medical field, the need for close

* Corresponding Author

assessment of the organs to be studied as well as the need for guidance of procedures under real time image. The first ultrasound tipped catheters were created to obtain organ dimensions and organ distances. No Doppler velocities or cross sectional images were obtained

In 1956, Cieszynsky et al. used the first ultrasound tip catheter in dogs; he found it to be useful without injury to the system being observed. In the mid-1960s, Kossofs et al used the first ICE in measuring the thickness of the ventricular septum and ventricular wall by M-mode with surprising precision, but the catheter lacked mobility when it was inside the heart. In 1969, a mechanically rotating 4-element probe was developed by Eggleton et al and during the same time the first two dimensional real time ultrasound tip catheter was developed by Bom et al.

In 1974 Reid introduced the Doppler system by measuring Doppler velocities of femoral and coronary artery in dogs and in 1975 Gichard et al developed a new concept of catheter in which the shaft was more flexible with the ability to rotate inside the heart.

In the mid-1980s, percutaneous transluminal coronary angioplasty was adopted in many centers as the procedure of choice for coronary artery disease. This advancement in the field of cardiac catheterization created the need for development of an ideal device for intracardiac echo. The goal was to create a catheter with a flexible shaft, predictable orientation inside the heart with lower frequency transducers, superior imaging depth as well as enhanced tissue penetration.

Pandian et al in 1990 used the ICE catheter for the first time in humans in detecting iliofemoral artery obstructing disease with the ability to distinguish diseased arteries from normal vessels. Subsequently he used ICE in guidance of PTCA with encouraging results.

ICE was introduced to the field of congenital structural heart disease when Valdez-Cruz et al in 1991 described successful results of percutaneous closure of atrial septal defect (ASD) under ICE guidance in piglets. Since then, the utility of ICE has expanded. Electrophysiology studies demanded more accurate assessments during and after ablation studies. The first ablation procedure described under ICE guidance was by Seward et al in 1996 in dogs; it was found to have more accurate assessment of the size of the ablation injury, enhanced visual detection of intramyocardial hematoma and thrombus formation which were not well seen by fluoroscopy or even by TEE.

In the subsequent years as we mentioned above, ICE has had a tremendous advancement in technology and it has been described to be useful in the guidance of most cardiac interventional procedures such as ASD/PFO/VSD device closure, balloon valvuloplasty, aortic coarctation angioplasty/stent placement or other central vascular stenosis, transeptal puncture, percutaneous pulmonary and aortic valve placement, left atrial appendage closure and many others.

3. ICE catheters

Over the past several years, improvements in technology have allowed the development of intracardiac transducers of lower frequency as well as Doppler imaging capability with improved depth penetration and better image resolution.

At present, there are five different transducer technologies for real-time intracardiac ultrasonic imaging

1. The *ultraICE* mechanical single-element system (Boston Scientific Corp, San Jose, CA, USA)
2. The *AcuNav* system from Siemens from Biosense-Webster
3. The *Clear ICE* system from St Jude Medical
4. The *SoundStar Catheter* system from Biosense-Webster
5. The *ViewMate Z* Intracardiac Ultrasound System and *ViewFlex Plus* ICE Catheter from St Jude Medical.

The UltraICE system (Boston Scientific Corp, San Jose, CA, USA) is a 9 MHz single element transducer incorporated in a 9F catheter. The catheter is not steerable and it lacks Doppler capabilities. This system provides cross-sectional images in a 360° radial plane with only 5 cms radial field depth which provides near-field clarity but poor tissue penetration; hence the left sided structures are not possible to obtained when the ultrasound catheter is in the Right heart. It has been used in guidance of coronary artery interventional procedures because of the catheter's capability of producing near - field images. Three-dimensional reconstruction of the anatomy can be obtained as well.

The ClearICE device (St. Jude Medical, Inc) has a 64-element phased-array transducer with a highly steerable catheter and bidirectional steering up to 140°. It works with the Vivid system (GE Healthcare Technologies, Wauwatosa, WI). It has two sets of electrodes for integration of 3D localization with NavX. Apart from grayscale and tissue Doppler; it also allows for synchronization mapping and 2D speckle tracking.

The SoundStar Catheter system (Biosense-Webster) has the same characteristics like AcuNav catheter but with CARTO magnetic sensor in the tip.

The ViewFlex Plus catheter (St. Jude Medical, Inc.) uses the ViewMate Z ultrasound system (EPMedSystems, Inc., Berlin, NJ). It has a 64-element phased-array transducer with a frequency of 4.5 to 8.5 MHz, and an imaging depth of 12 cm. it has a steerable catheter via two-way articulation; it can be rotated axially and steered in anterior and posterior directions up to 120° with enhanced tip stability. It also allows a two-way flex color Doppler and grayscale. This catheter has the ability to quickly produce exceptional images in a compact, cart-based system.

Currently AcuNav catheter (Biosense Webster, Inc, Diamond Bar, CA, USA) (FIGURE 1) is the most popular ICE catheter used for guidance of percutaneous closure of an ASD. The catheter size decreased from 11F to 8 F in diameter in the last years and now requires only an 8 Fr introducer with subsequent fewer traumas to the vessel entered. The catheter consists of a miniaturized 64-element phased-array transducer with color, tissue and spectral Doppler capabilities; the frequency of the transducer varies from 5.5 to 10 MHz and it provides a 90° sector image with excellent tissue penetration up to 16 cm for the 8F catheter, allowing visualization of left-sided structures from the right heart. The catheter is somewhat stiff but with a brilliant four-way articulation that provides excellent maneuverability inside the heart; the handle has a locking knob that allows the catheter tip to be fixed in a desired position. This is an important feature of this catheter. It works with Sequoia, Cypress, or Aspen imaging systems, all of which are manufactured by Siemens Medical Solutions USA, Inc. (Malvern, PA). It can be introduced by a femoral or internal jugular approach; The 8 F catheter is 90-110 cms long and careful advancement from the groin to the heart under continuous fluoroscopic guidance is recommended, unless a long sheath (>30 cms) is used in the femoral vein.

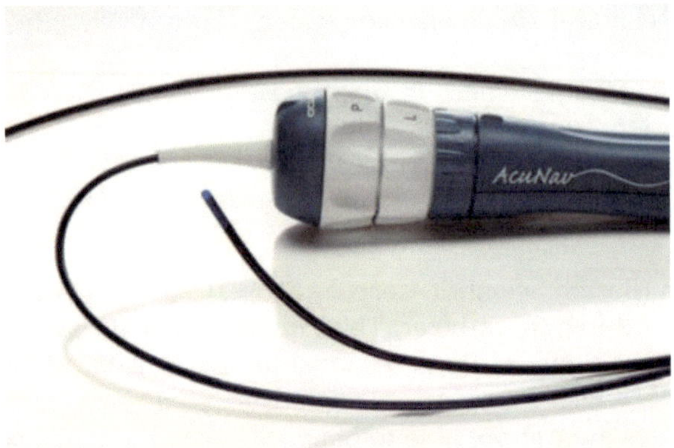

Fig. 1. AcuNav Catheter; the control handle has three knobs: one to move the tip in posterior/anterior directions, one to move the tip in right/left directions, and the last knob is a locking one that will fix the tip in the desired orientation.

4. ICE catheter insertion techniques

The catheter can be introduced by femoral or internal jugular approach; however the femoral vein approach is the most popular among most of the interventionalists because it is closer to the table, allowing easier manipulation of the control handle. The 8 F AcuNav catheter is 90-110 cms long and careful advancement from the groin to the heart under continuous fluoroscopic guidance is recommended because of its rigidity (stiffness) and possible advancement of the catheter into side branches with potential vessel injury before reaching the right atrium (RA); it is recommended to use a long 8 french sheath (30 cms) in either femoral vein in order to avoid vascular complications or possibly entanglement below the level of the IVC. This approach offers easy accessibility and allows fairly free movement of the catheter inside the heart. In adult patients, the catheter can be introduced in the same vein used for the device delivery (FIGURE 2). For patients with weight below 35 kg, access in the opposite femoral vein is recommended (FIGURE 2).

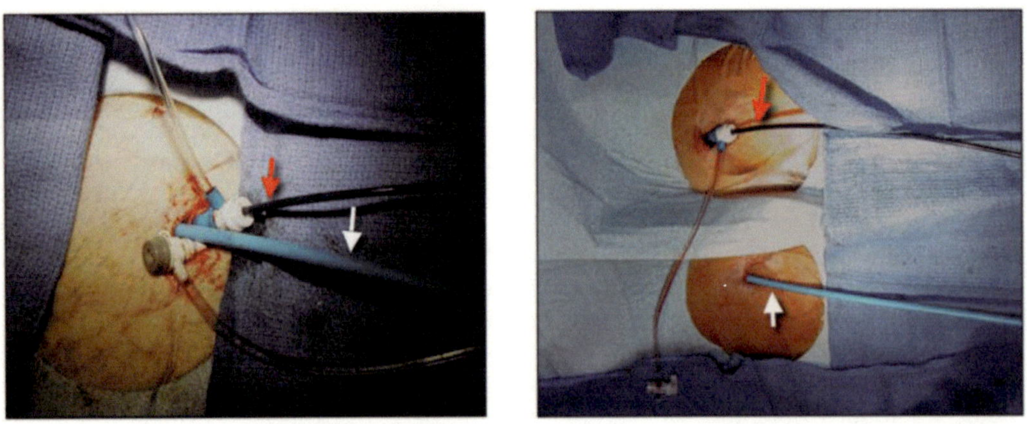

Fig. 2. ICE catheter insertion; Left: Adult patient with ICE catheter (red arrow) and delivery sheath (white arrow) in same femoral vein. Right: Pediatric patient with ICE catheter (red arrow) and delivery sheath (white arrow) in opposite veins.

The superior vena cava (SVC) is another option to achieve access to the RA. This approach can be accomplished either from the right internal jugular vein or the left subclavian vein into the RA.

5. ICE guidance protocol for ASD closure

The ICE catheter is introduced in the usual fashion and advanced from the inferior vena cava (IVC) into the RA. We start the ICE protocol obtaining first the home view, septal view, long axis view and short axis view in combination with fluoroscopic image (FIGURE 3).

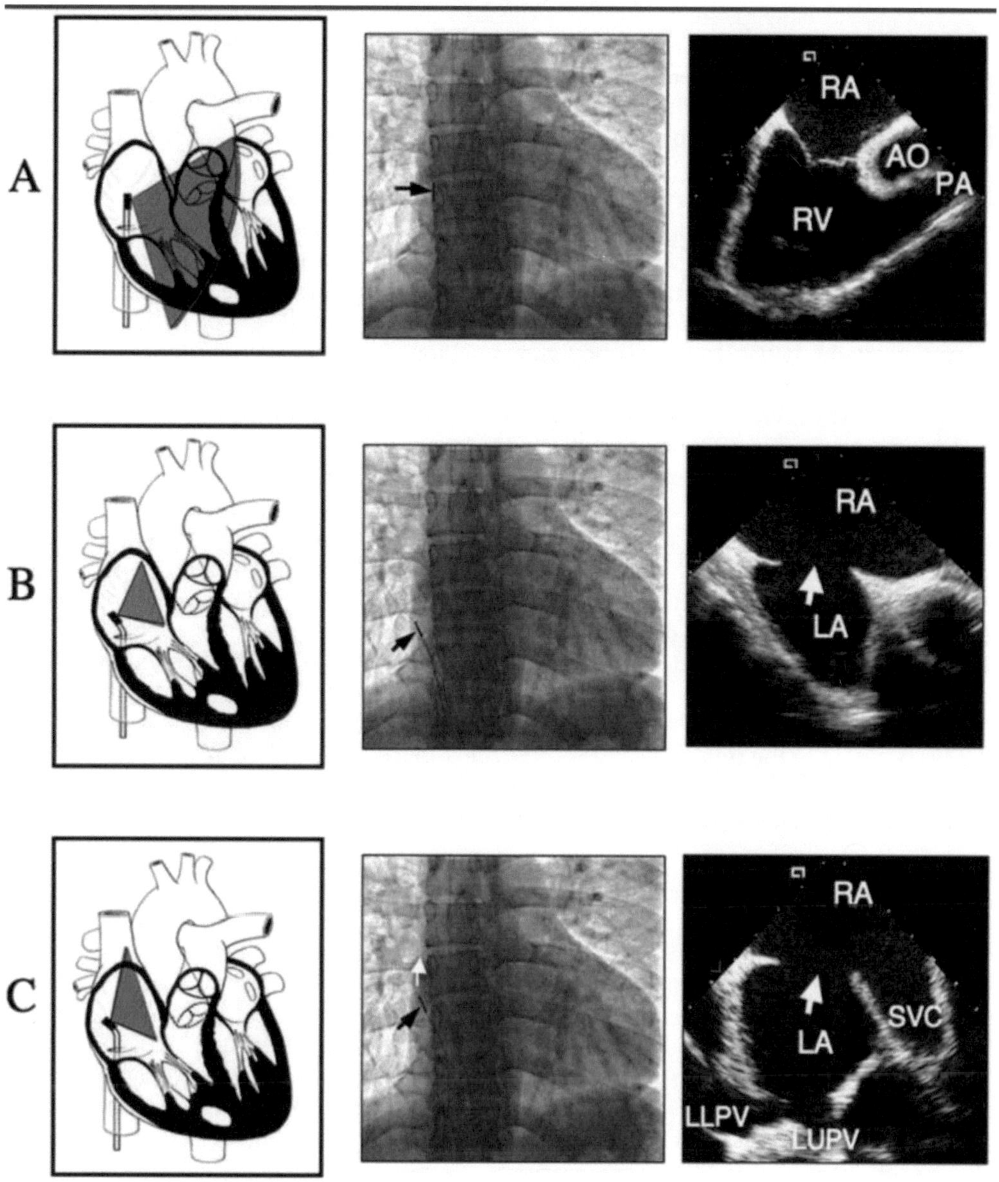

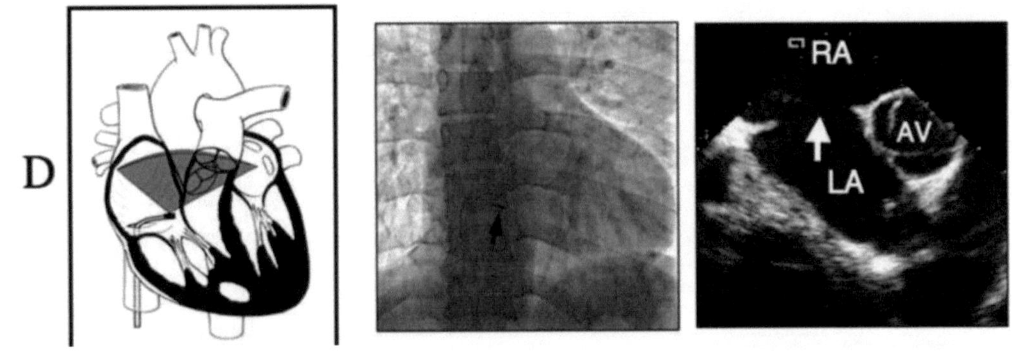

Fig. 3. Fluoroscopy and ICE assesment of an ASD; (A) Home view. Left, heart diagram with the position of the ICE catheter in the neutral 'home view' position. The shaded area represents structures seen in this view. Middle, A-P Fluoroscopic image of the ICE catheter positioned in the mid RA (arrow) and parallel to the spine. Right, ICE 2-D image in the neutral home view position. The tricuspid valve, right atrium (RA), right ventricle (RV), RV outflow tract, pulmonary artery (PA) and aorta in short axis are well seen in this position. (B) Septal view. Left, heart diagram with the position of the ICE catheter in the posterior flexed position looking at the atrial septum 'septal view'. The shaded area represents structures seen in this view. Middle, Fluoroscopic A-P image of the ICE catheter (arrow) in the RA pointing to the right side of the heart and the transducer flexed posterior looking at the septum. Right, ICE 2-D image septal view position. The right atrium (RA), left atrium (LA) and the atrial septal defect are well seen (arrow) in this position.
(C) Long-axis 'caval view'. Left, heart diagram with the position of the ICE catheter in the posterior flexed position with a more superior advancement looking at the atrial septum and the superior vena cava. The shaded area represents structures seen in this view. Middle, A-P Fluoroscopic image of the ICE catheter (black arrow) demonstrating catheter pointing posteriorly to the septum and positioned higher than the septal view closer to the SVC (white arrow). Right, ICE 2-D image in the long axis view position. The atrial septal defect (arrow), right atrium (RA), left atrium (LA), left upper, left lower pulmonary veins (LUPV, LLPV), and the superior vena cava (SVC) are all well seen.
(D) Short-axis view. Left, heart diagram with the position of the ICE catheter in the flexed position but now positioned near the tricuspid valve and below the aortic valve. The shaded area represents structures seen in this view. Middle, Fluoroscopic A-P image of the ICE catheter pointing to the right side of the spine, next to the tricuspid valve and just below the aortic valve. Right, ICE 2-D image in the short-axis view. The atrial septal defect (arrow), the left atria (LA), right atria (RA) and the aortic valve are all well seen in this view.

5.1 Standard views

5.1.1 Home view

This view can be obtained by advancing the ICE catheter to the mid right atrium. Catheter is parallel to the spine with the transducer portion facing the tricuspid valve. Subtle counter clockwise movements in the knob of the catheter can be done to obtain the home view image. When you are in home view you should see the right atrium, the tricuspid valve, the right ventricle, right ventricular inflow and outflow and a portion of the aortic valve in short axis view. The anterior portion of the septum can be occasionally visualized as well. (FIGURE 4).

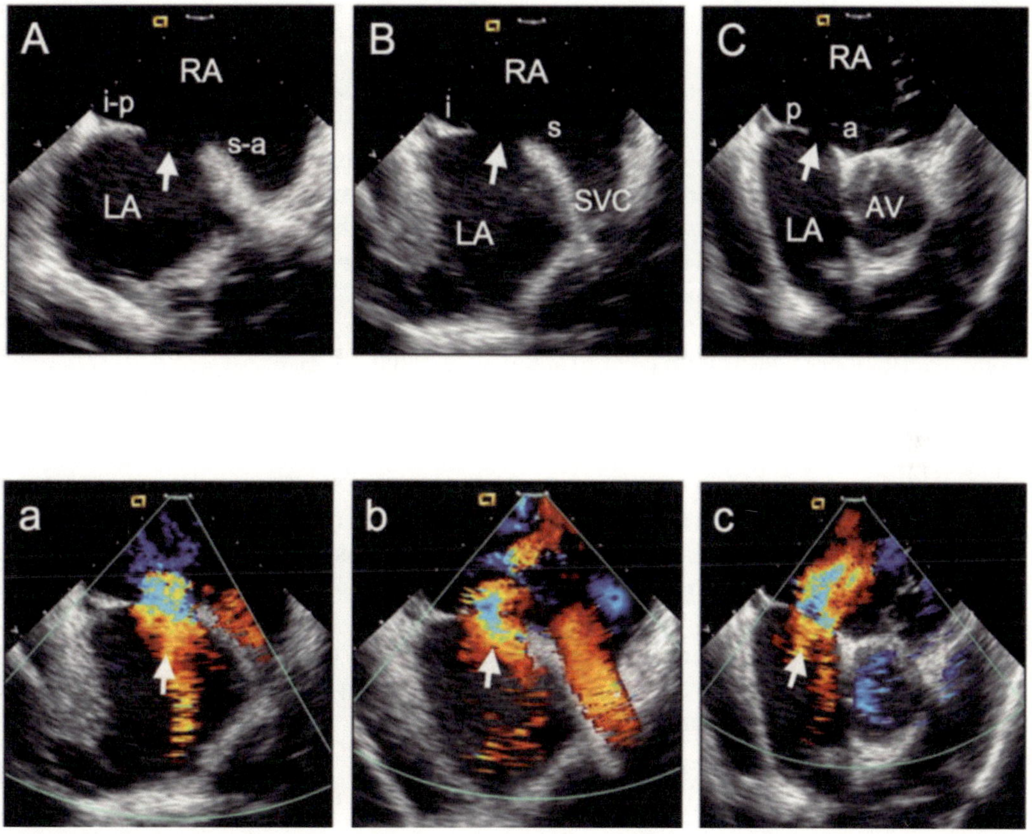

Fig. 4. Septal View: Left A) ICE 2-D image demonstrating a large ASD (arrow), right atrium (RA), left atrium (LA), the superior anterior rim (s-a) and the inferior posterior rim (i-p) a) ICE color image demonstrating a large ASD (arrow) with left to right shunt. Long axis view: Center B) ICE 2-D image demonstrating large ASD (arrow), superior vena cava (SVC) right atrium (RA), left atrium (LA), superior rim (s) and inferior rim (i). b) ICE color image showing a large ASD (arrow) with left to right shunt and SVC drainage to RA. Short Axis View: Right C) ICE 2-D image demonstrating a large ASD (arrow), right atrium (RA), left atrium (LA), aortic valve (AV), anterior rim (a) and posterior rim (p). c) ICE color image showing a large atrial septal defect with left to right shunt.

5.1.2 Septal view

After the home view image is obtained, slight movements of the anterior-posterior knob posteriorly and the right-left knob rightward will make the transducer face the atrial septum. In this view you can see the entire length of the atrial septum. The image closer to the ICE catheter (superior) is the RA and distal to the image (inferior) is the left atrium.

Occasionally you can see the pulmonary venous return to the left atrium and the coronary sinus as well. Once you lock the catheter you can make fine movements in the knob or rotate the entire catheter to get the image that suits better guidance of the procedure. (FIGURE 4)

5.1.3 Long axis view

This view can be obtained after having the catheter in the septal view, followed by slight superior advancement of the ICE catheter in the RA towards the SVC. The catheter can either face the atrial septum, the SVC or both; it depends on the position of the catheter. Advancing the flexed catheter in the direction of the SVC can profile much better the SVC and the respective posterior superior rim. Withdrawal of the flexed catheter towards the IVC will profile the inferior part of the atrial septum and the posterior inferior rim as well. This view is good for measurements of an atrial septal defect as well. The right and left pulmonary venous drainage can be seen just rotating the catheter clockwise or counterclockwise as well as with flexion/anteflexion. (FIGURE 4).

5.1.4 Short axis view

The catheter is still flexed in its locked position; to obtain the image, the entire catheter should be moved from the sheath hub in a clockwise manner in order to place it inferior to the aortic valve and near the tricuspid valve; this is followed by slight adjustments in the posterior anterior knob with less posterior flexion and more leftward rotation on the right/left knob. Fluoroscopy image shows the position of the catheter. This view is the opposite of the short axis view that can be obtained using TEE with the near field image being the right atrium and the far field image being the left atrium. The superior anterior rim and inferoposterior rim can be obtained as well (FIGURE 4).

5.2 ICE guidance during and after device deployment

5.2.1 The defect is crossed with a wire; this image is crucial in complex atrial septal defects or fenestrated ASD's to confirm that the largest defect is being crossed by the wire. Subsequently the delivery sheath is advanced and placed in one of the left pulmonary veins (Figure 5)

5.2.2 Balloon sizing is also of significant importance in large or complex defects for further delineation of the atrial septal defect (FIGURE 6) and to measure the "stop-flow diameter" of the defect.

5.2.3 The device is advanced and the left disk deployed in the left atrium and positioned in a way that is oriented with the atrial septum. The left disk is slowly pulled back to the atrial septum. The device position is constantly evaluated by ICE, making sure its position in relation to the left side of the atrium is maintained. When the device makes contact with the defect; it is important well seated; it makes good well seated; makes good contact with all available rims and the left disk doesn't protrude to the RA . this is followed by deployment of the right atrial disk in the right atrium. Deployment of the device is always done under fluoroscopic and ICE guidance for successful results (FIGURE 7A-7B)

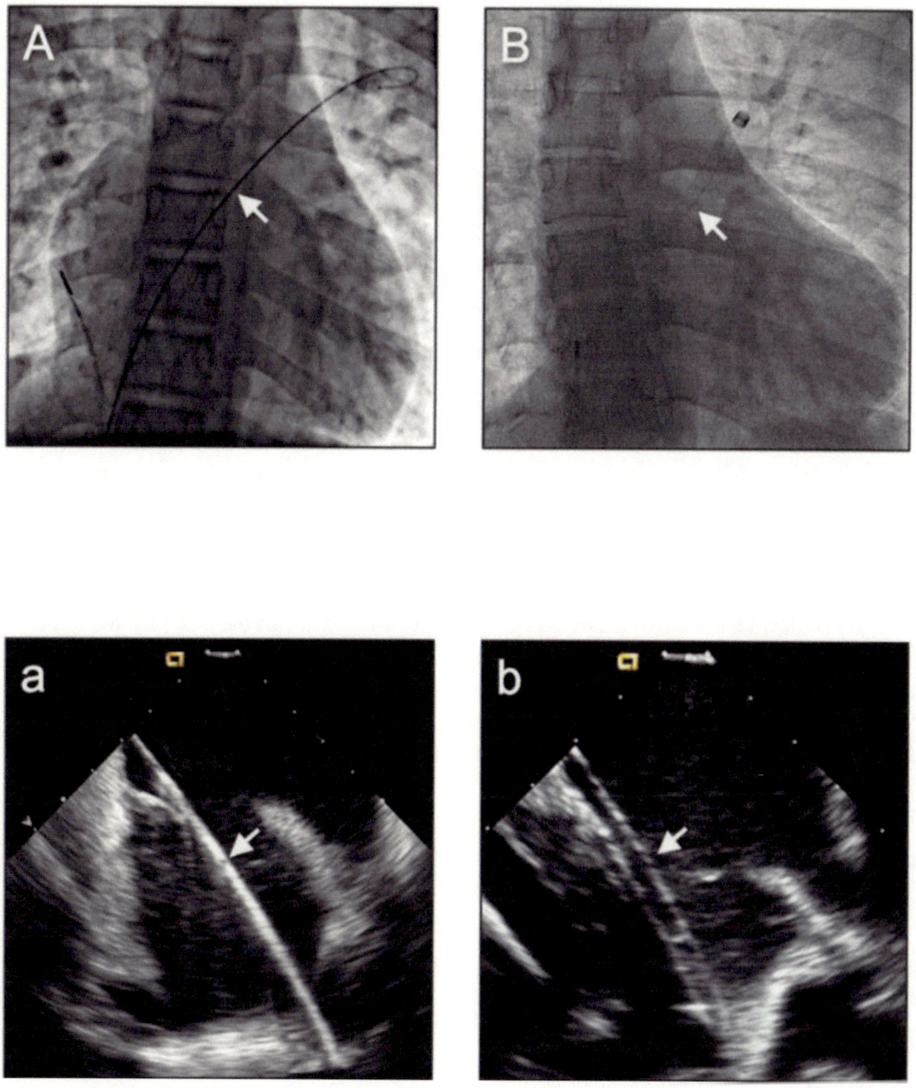

Fig. 5. Wire and delivery sheath assessment. Left A) A-P fluoroscopic image of the wire (arrow) crossing the ASD and positioned in the left upper pulmonary septal view demonstrating the wire (arrow) crossing the large ASD and the tip located in the left upper pulmonary vein. Right B) fluoroscopic image showing sheath (arrow) crossing the ASD and positioned in the left upper pulmonary vein. b) ICE septal view demonstrating the sheath (arrow) crossing the ASD and positioned in the left upper pulmonary vein.

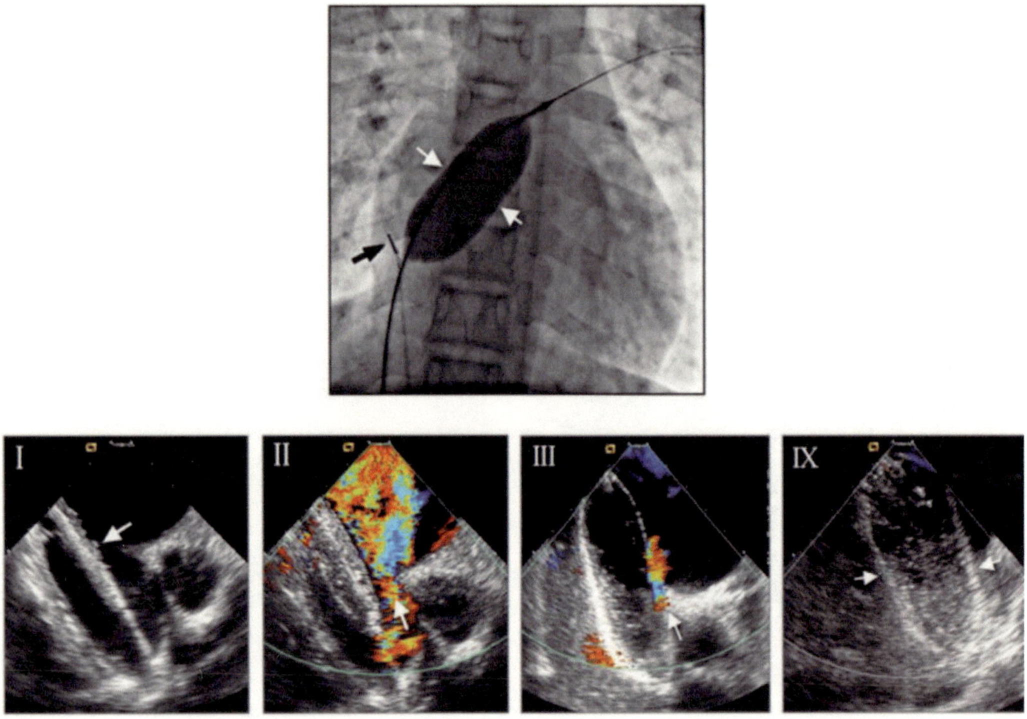

Fig. 6. Balloon "Stop-flow" diameter assessment; . I) Balloon sizing deflated (arrow) crossing the ASD. II) Balloon inflated with evidence of residual shunt (arrow). III) Balloon inflated again with evidence of very mild residual shunt (arrow). IV) Balloon stop flow diameter (white arrows) achieved without evidence of residual shunt. Image in top demonstrating an A-P fluoroscopic image of the stop flow balloon sizing diameter (white arrows), ICE catheter (black arrow) positioned in the septal view during balloon inflation.

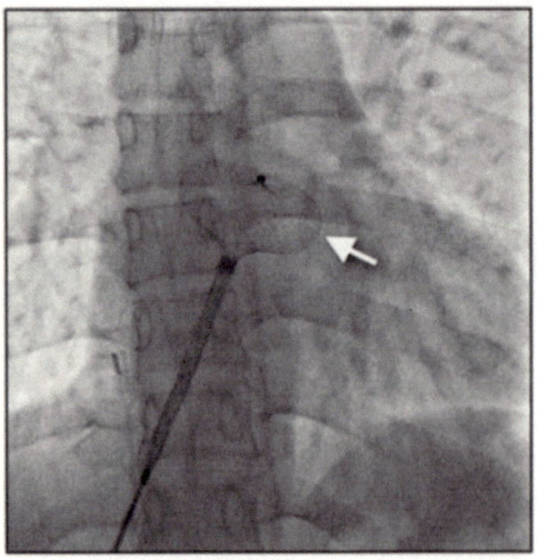

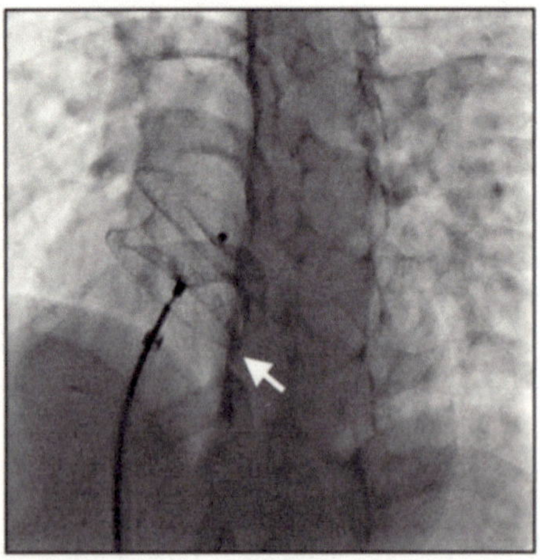

Fig. 7A. Left and right atrial Disks Deployment. Left) Fluoroscopic image of the left atrial disk (arrow) deployed in the LA. Right) A-P Fluoroscopic image in the hepatoclavicular view demonstrating the right atrial disk (arrow) deployed in the RA.

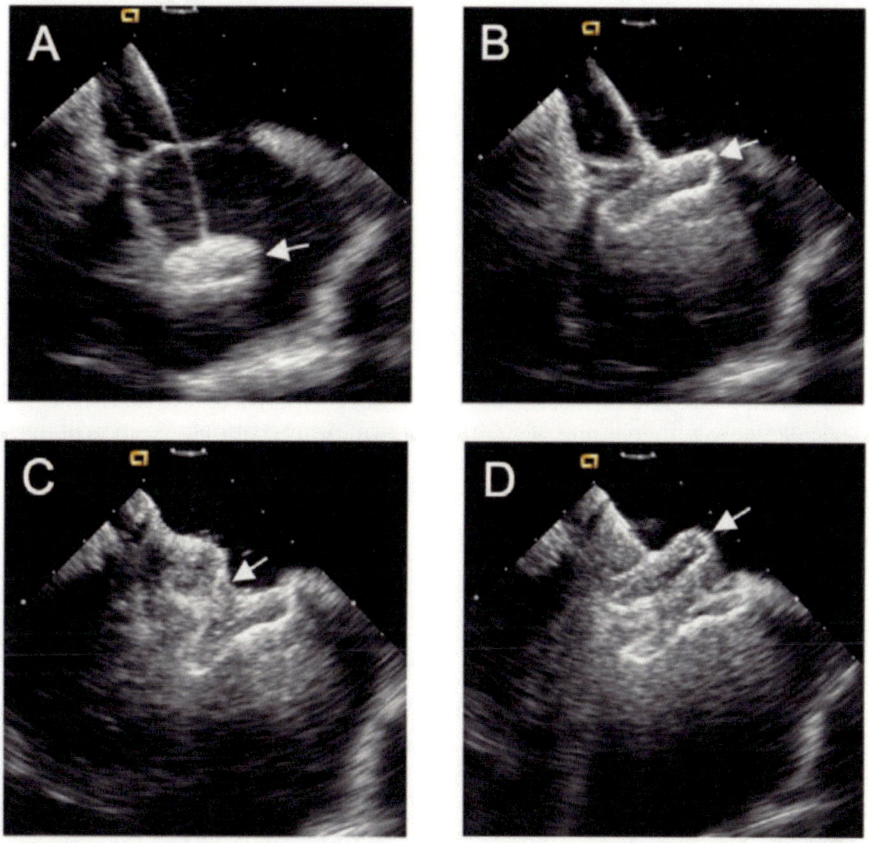

Fig. 7B. A) ICE image in short axis view demonstrating the left atrial disk (arrow) deployed in left atrium in alignment with the ASD. B) Continuous ICE assessment in septal view of the left disk while is pulled back to the left side of superior and inferior posterior rims. C) ICE image in septal view demonstrating the waist of the device (arrow) before complete deployment of right disk D) ICE image in septal view demonstrating the deployment of right atrial disk (arrow).

5.2.4 After right disk is deployed, subsequent assessment of the position and stability of the device is done. Long axis view view and short axis view are the best views for assessment of the device position prior to its release. Assessment of device stability, residual shunt , SVC and IVC is important before releasing the device. Again fluoroscopic image correlation with ICE images is essential for assessment of device position and stability before releasing the device (FIGURE 8A-8B).

5.2.5 After releasing the device, further assessment for device stability is performed with fluoroscopy and ICE; Evaluation of nearby structures and assessment of any residual shunt is done again in short axis, septal and long axis views (FIGURE 9A-9B).

It is very important to remember that before pulling out the ICE catheter from the sheath, it must be unlocked before withdrawal to the IVC.

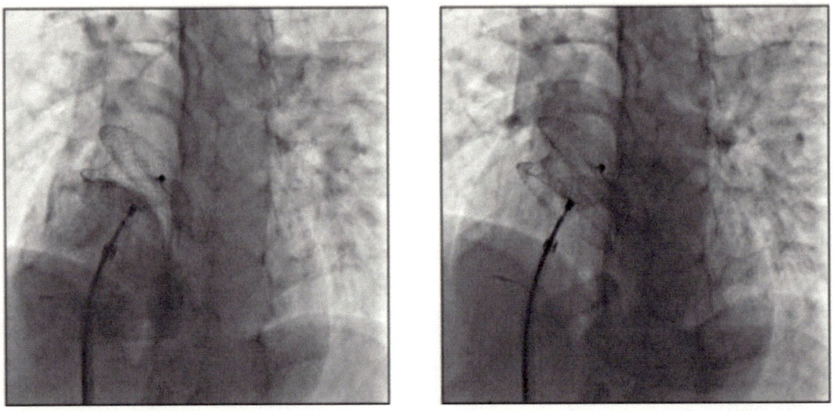

Fig. 8A. Fluoroscopic pre-release assessment of device. A) Fluoroscopic image in the hepatoclavicular view with injection of contrast confirming appropriate position of the right atrial disk in the atrial septum. B) Fluoroscopic image in the hepatoclavicular view with contrast on levophase confirming appropriate position of the left atrial disk in the atrial septum.

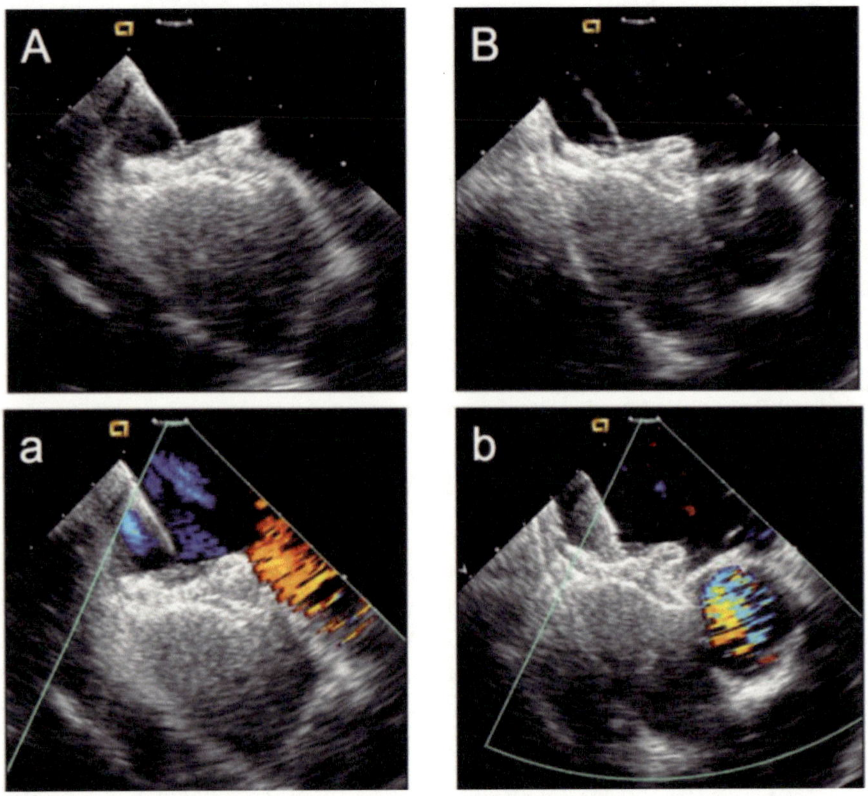

Fig. 8B. ICE pre-release assessment of device. A) ICE 2-D image in long axis view demonstrating the device well seated.a) ICE with color in long axis view demonstrating normal SVC flow and no residual shunt; delivery system still attached to the device. B) ICE 2-D image in short axis view demonstrating the device well seated. b)ICE with color in short axis view demonstrating no residual shunt.

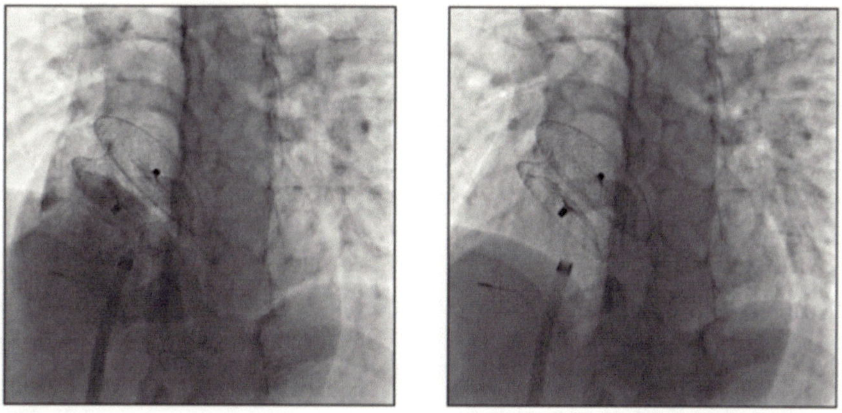

Fig. 9A. Fluoroscopic final assessment: Left) Fluoroscopic image in the hepatoclavicular view confirming device not attached to the delivery system and after contrast Injection, right atrial disk appeared to be in good position. Right) Fluoroscopic image with injection of contrast on levophase confirmed appropriate positioned of the left atrial disk after being released from the delivery system.

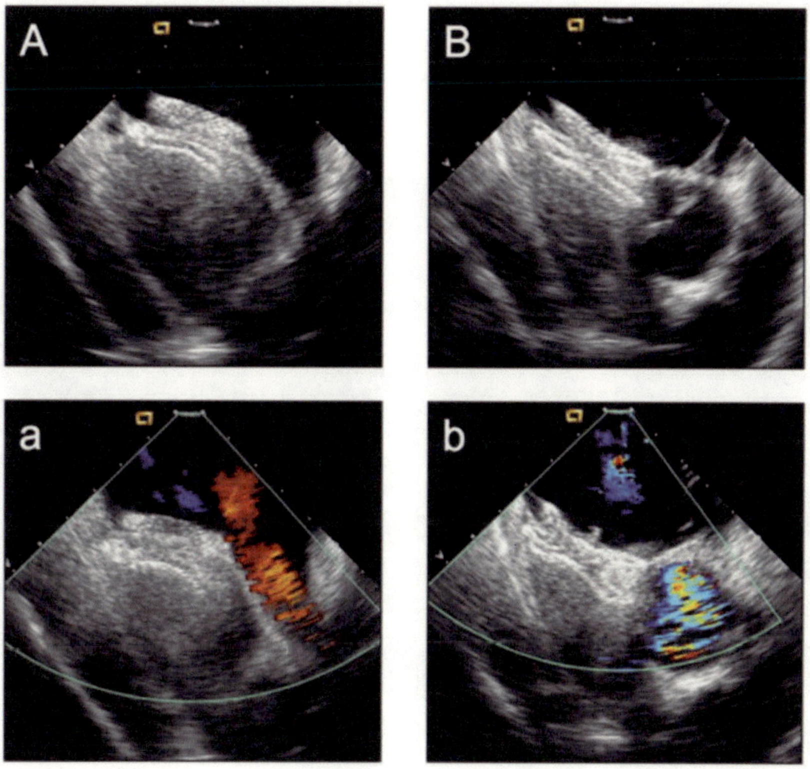

Fig. 9B. ICE final assessment post release of device: A) ICE 2-D image in long axis view demonstrating the device well seated. a) ICE with color in long axis view demonstrating normal SVC flow and no residual shunt. B) ICE 2-D image in short axis view demonstrating the device well seated. b) ICE with color in short axis view demonstrating no residual shunt.

6. Advantages and limitations of ICE

Transthoracic Echocardiogram (TTE) has been used for guidance of percutaneous closure of ASDs. However the pictures sometimes are not accurate to evaluate the size of the defect and it is difficult for evaluation of the rims, therefore risking stability of the device. Further, due to it being close to the working area of the intervention, there is risk to compromise sterility of the procedure. The advantages are that it can be done under conscious sedation and it is cheaper than ICE and TEE.

The use of TEE is well known for guidance of percutaneous closure of ASDs. It provides excellent intracardiac resolution and has 3D capabilities. However, it requires sedation and possible endotracheal intubation, it is uncomfortable for patients, and may raise the cost of the procedure due to professional and procedural fees.

ICE has been used in the last decade for guidance of percutaneous closure of ASDs and is lately gaining more acceptance in the interventional community. It provides excellent real time cardiac resolution as good as or even superior to TEE without exposing patients to the risks of deep sedation or endotracheal intubation. Several studies have shown decrease in fluoroscopy time, interventional procedure time, and catheterization laboratory time when compared with TEE and subsequent decrease in radiation exposure and procedure cost.

ICE has the advantage of having an accurate evaluation of all ASDs as compared to TEE which sometimes can miss an inferior-posterior atrial septal defect (FIGURE 10A, 10B, 10C). It is also important in the evaluation of fenestrated ASDs by determining the larger defect and this allows accurate evaluation of the larger defect while it is being crossed by a wire and during balloon sizing (FIGURE 11).

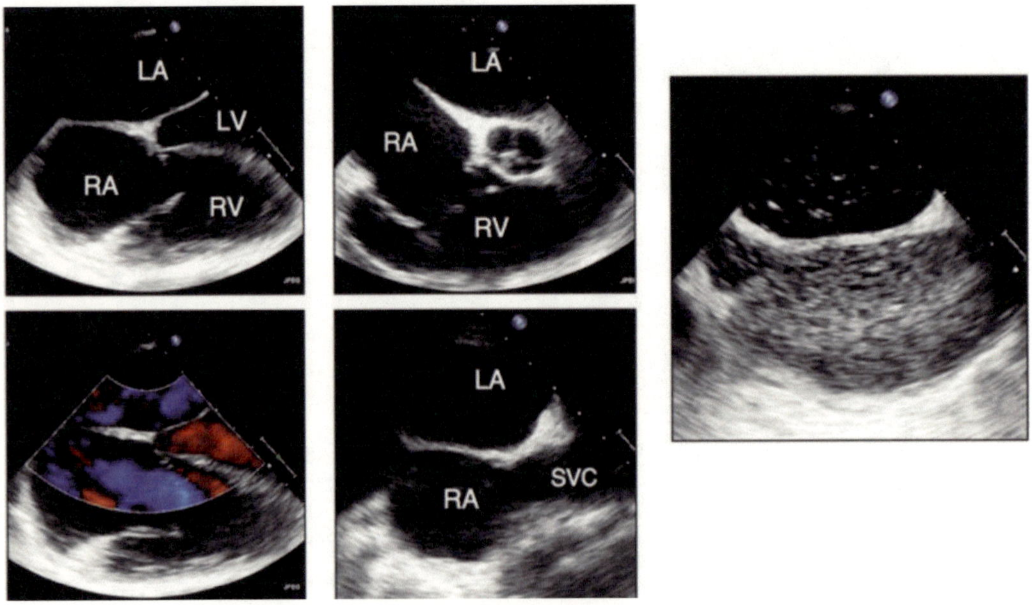

Fig. 10A. Inferior posterior ASD missed with TEE. TEE in four chamber, short axis and long axis view demonstrating intact atrial septum by 2-D and by color. Figure to the right demonstrating positive bubble study when injected in the right atrium. Right Atrium RA, Left Atrium LA, Right Ventricle RV, Left Ventricle LV, Superior vena Cava SVC.

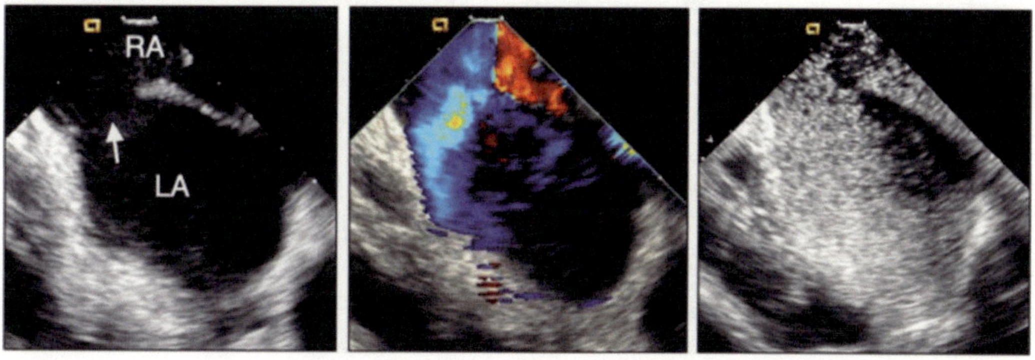

Fig. 10B. Inferior posterior ASD detected with ICE. Modified septal view showed small inferior posterior atrial septal defect (arrow) and confirmed with bubbles from the RA to the LA. Right atrium RA, Left atrium LA.

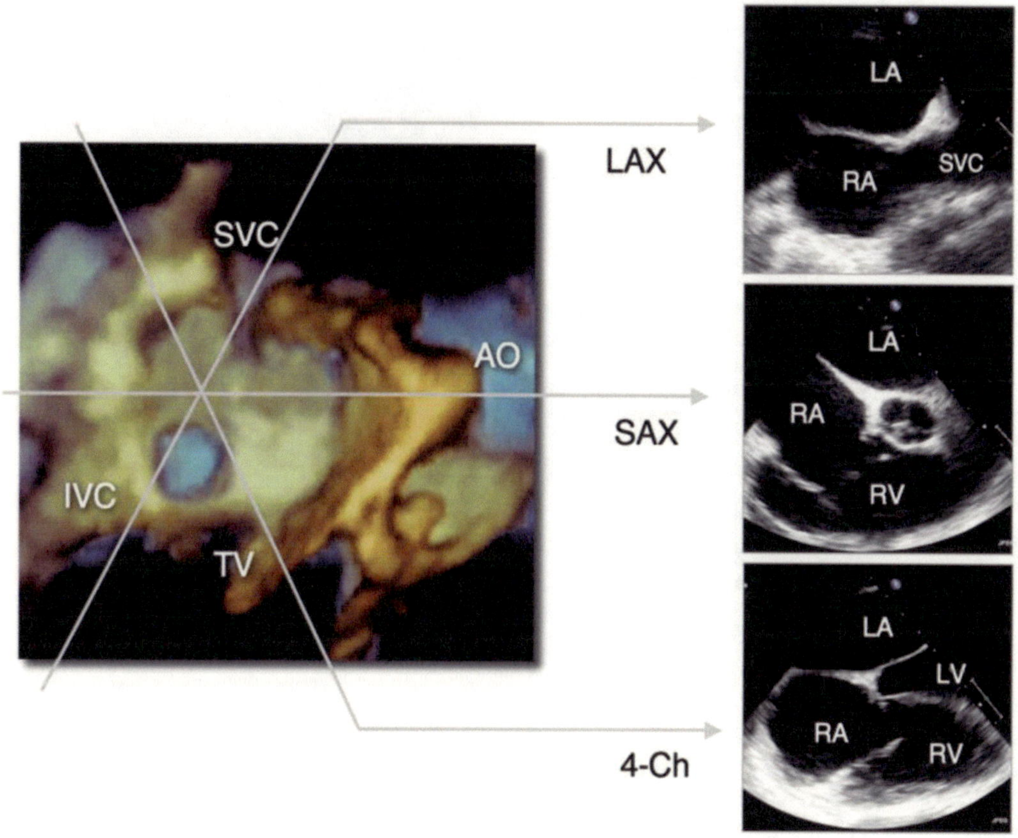

Fig. 10C. TEE 3-D. Left) TEE detected small inferior posterior defect by 3D; Right) Demonstrating different cuts while performing standard TEE 2-D views and how an inferior posterior atrial defect can be missed if 3-D image is not performed.

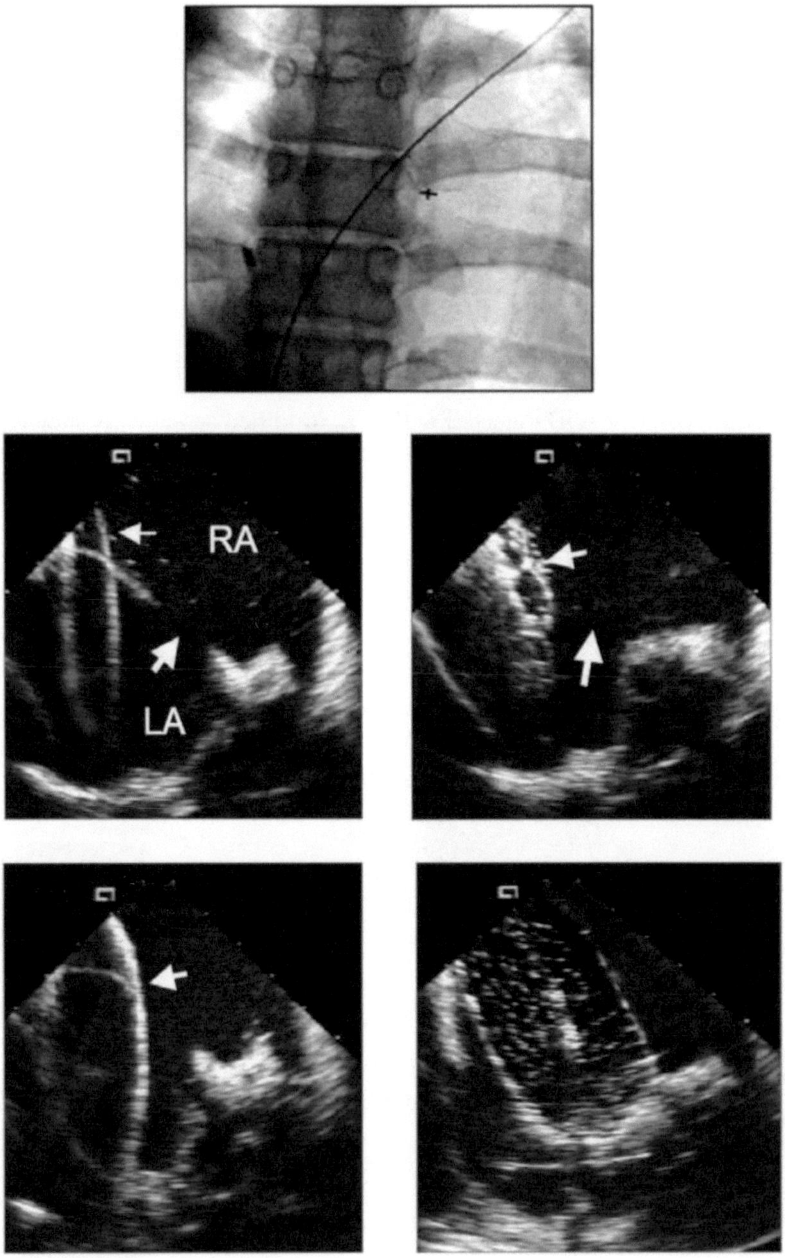

Fig. 11. Fenestrated ASD assessment. ICE images to the left demonstrating fenestrated ASD crossed by a wire (arrow). Larger atrial septal defect (arrow) not crossed by the wire. Subsequent balloon partially inflated with waist (arrow), confirming smaller atrial septal defect crossed by the wire. ICE images to the bottom demonstrating correct position of the wire crossing larger defect with successful balloon stop flow diameter. Fluoroscopic image in the top demonstrating wire crossing atrial septal defect and positioned in the left upper pulmonary vein.

The limitations of ICE include its large shaft size (8 French), and cost. In addition, there is no real time three-dimensional (3D) available in the market yet.

7. Complications related to ICE catheter

At the present time only vascular complications have been reported in the literature. There are some potential complications that may result from ICE and these are the same as the ones being reported during right heart catheterization. Transient arrhythmias can result from direct contact of the probe to the wall of the chamber. The arrhythmia should disappear after adjusting the position of the catheter. Thrombus formation around the catheter can also happen during any intracardiac procedure but can be prevented with adequate anticoagulation and decreasing the time of the ICE catheter inside the body. Other potential complications such as pericardial tamponade, pulmonary embolism, and bleeding/infection from the puncture site are infrequent but can occur as well.

8. Conclusion

ICE has shown to be helpful in guiding cardiac catheter interventions, especially EP studies and transcatheter closure of ASDs.

The use of ICE is becoming more popular for guidance of interventional procedures, especially for ASD closure (evaluation of the defect and rims and live guidance during device deployment). It has also been found to be extremely helpful during guidance of closure of complex atrial septal defects.

Currently ICE systems are easily available in the market; the skills in maneuvering the catheter and interpreting the images are not difficult to learn. The real time structural and hemodynamic information are comparable or even better than TEE with an accurate and safe procedural guidance for transcatheter closure of ASDs. The capabilities of identifying complications immediately during the procedure are exceptional.

So far to our knowledge there are no major complication reported and the only minor complications that can be encountered are related to the site of access and during advancement of the catheter. Although the risk potential seems to be low, it is mandatory that the ICE catheter is handled with caution, since it is not wire-guided.

Because the ICE catheter is inserted through the femoral vein, similar to other cardiac catheters; it allows the interventionist to perform procedures without general anesthesia, shortening procedure time, and reducing fluoro exposure with subsequent reduction of radiation exposure and costs in personnel and equipment. There is no need of an extra skilled person for the TEE, and, as such, fewer physicians are required to be present for the procedure. This results in a shorter turnaround time in the cardiac catheterization laboratory.

In the future, the development of smaller and softer catheters will decrease the incidence of vascular complications. It may also be possible for the ICE catheter to be used in all pediatric age groups. Three-dimensional/four dimensional real time images are not so far away from being developed and an extraordinary understanding of the intracardiac anatomy during any intracardiac procedure will be achieved. Advancement of guidewires, catheters and devices through the ICE catheter can potentially be available as well.

Along with fluoroscopy it is likely that ICE will improve the safety and outcome of percutaneous closure of ASDs. With all its inherent advantages, ICE may soon replace TEE as a guiding tool not only in adults but also in adolescents and children

9. References

Alboliras ET & Hijazi ZM: Comparison of costs of intracardiac echocardiography and transesophageal echocardiography in monitoring percutaneous device closure of atrial septal defect in children and adults. Am J Cardiol 2004; 94:690-692

Amin Z, Cao QL & Hijazi ZM: Intracardiac echocardiography for structural lesions. Card Intervent Today 2009, April/May

Awad S, Cao QL & Hijazi ZM: Intracardiac echocardiography for the guidance of percutaneous procedures. Curr Cardiol Reports 2009, 11:210-215

Bom N, Lancee CT & Van Egmond FC: An ultrasonic intracardiac scanner. Ultrasonics.1972; 10: 72-76.

Bom N, ten Hoff & Lancee CT: Early and recent intraluminal ultrasound devices. Int J Cardiac Imaging.1989; 4: 79-88

Bruce CJ, Packer DL & Belohlavek M: Intracardiac echocardiography: newest technology. J Am Soc Echocardiogr. 2000; 13:788 -795.

Bruce CJ, Packer DL & Belohlavek M: Intracardiac echocardiography: newest technology. J Am Soc Echocardiogr. 2000; 13:788 -795.

Bruce CJ, Nishimura RA & Rihal CS et al: Intracardiac echocardiography in the interventional catheterization laboratory: preliminary experience with a novel, phased-array transducer. Am J Cardiol 2002; 89(5): 635–40.

Cao QL, Zabal C & Koenig P et al: Initial clinical experience with intracardiac echocardiography in guiding transcatheter closure of perimembranous ventricular septal defects: Feasibility and comparison with transesophageal echocardiography. Catheter Cardiovasc Intervent 2005; 66:258-267

Chen C, Guerrero JL & Vazquez de Prada JA et al. Intracardiac ultrasound measurement of volumes and ejection fraction in normal, infarcted, and aneurysmal left ventricles using a 10-MHz ultrasound catheter. Circ 1994; 90(3): 1481–91

Daoud EG, Kalbfleisch SJ & Hummel JD: Intracardiac echocardiography to guide transeptal left heart catheterization for radiofrequency catheter ablation. J Cardiovasc Electrophysiol.1999; 10(3): 358–63.

Eggleton RC, Townsend C & Kossoff G: Computerized ultrasonic visualization of dynamic ventricular configuration. In: Program and Abstracts of the Eighth ICBME; Palmer House, Chicago, Ill; July 1969; session 10-3.

Hijazi ZM, Cao, QL & Heitschmidt M: Catheter closure of multiple atrial septal defects under intracardiac echocardiographic guidance in a child using the Amplatzer Septal Occluder. Acunav Case Study Report for Acuson, 2001.

Hijazi ZM, Cao QL & Heitschmidt M et al: Residual inferior atrial septal defect after surgical repair: Closure under intracardiac echocardiographic guidance. J Invasiv Card 2001; 13:810-813

Hijazi ZM, Wang Z & Cao QL et al: Transcatheter closure of atrial septal defects and patent foramen ovale under intracardiac echocardiographic guidance: Feasibility and comparison with transesophageal echocardiography. Cath Cardiovasc Intervent 2001; 52:194-199

Hijazi ZM & Cao, QL: Transcatheter closure of secundum atrial septal defect associated with deficient posterior rim in a child under intracardiac echocardiographic guidance. Applications in Cardiac Imaging (Supplement of Applied Radiology), Nov 2002; 7-10

Hijazi ZM, Shivkumar K & Sahn DJ: Intracardiac echocardiography during interventional and electrophysiological cardiac catheterization. Circulation 2009, 119: 587-596

Kim S, Hijazi ZM & Lang RM et al: The use of intracardiac echocardiography and other intracardiac imaging tools to guide noncoronary cardiac interventions. J Amer Coll Cardiol 2009, 53:2117-2128

Koenig PK, Cao QL & Heitschmidt M et al: Role of intracardiac echocardiographic guidance in transcatheter closure of atrial septal defects and patent foramen ovale using the Amplatzer device. J Interven Cardiol 2003; 16:51-62

Koenig PR, Abdulla R & Cao QL et al: Use of intracardiac echocardiography to guide catheter closure of atrial communications. Echocardiography 2003; 20:781-787

Luxenberg DM, Silvestry FE & Herrmann HC et al: Use of a new 8French intracardiac echocardiographic catheter to guide device closure of atrial septal defects and patent foramen ovale in small children and adults: Initial clinical experience. J Invasive Cardiol 2005; 17:540-544

Mitchel JF, Gillam LD & Sanzobrono BW et al: Intracardiac ultrasound imaging during transeptal catheterization. Chest 1995; 108(1): 104–8.

Pandian NG, Kreis A, Brockway B et al: Ultrasound angioscopy: real-time, two-dimensional, intraluminal ultrasound imaging of blood vessels. Am J Cardiol. 1988 Sep 1;62(7):493-4

Pandian NG: Intravascular and intracardiac ultrasound imaging. An old concept, now on the road to reality. Circulation 1989, 80:1091-1094.

Ricou F, Ludomirsky A, Weintraub RG et al: Applications of intravascular scanning and transesophageal echocardiography in congenital heart disease: tradeoffs and the merging of technologies. Int J Card Imaging. 1991;6(3-4):221-30

Rigatelli G & Hijazi ZM: Intracardiac echocardiography in cardiovascular catheter-bases interventions: Different devices for different purposes. J Invas Cardiol 2006; 18:225-232

Tardif JC, Vannan MA & Miller DS et al: Potential applications of intracardiac echocardiography in interventional electrophysiology. Am Heart J 1994; 127(4 Pt 2): 1090–4.

Tardiff JC, Groenveld PW & Wang PJ et al. Intracardiac echocardiographic guidance during microwave catheter ablation. J Am Soc Echocardiogr 1999; 12(1): 41–7.

Valdes-Cruz LM, Sideris E, Sahn DJ et al: Transvascular intracardiac applications of a miniaturized phased-array ultrasonic endoscope. Initial experience with intracardiac imaging in piglets. Circulation. 1991 Mar;83(3):1023-7

Schwartz SL, Gillam LD & Weintraub AR et al: Intracardiac echocardiography in humans using a small-sized (6F), low frequency (12.5 MHz) ultrasound catheter: methods, imaging planes and clinical experience. J Am Coll Cardiol 1993; 21:189.

Section 5

ASD Closure in Adults and Elderly

8

Why, When and How Should Atrial Septal Defects Be Closed in Adults

P. Syamasundar Rao
University of Texas at Houston Medical School, Houston, TX, USA

1. Introduction

The most common defects in the atrial septum are ostium secundum, ostium primum and sinus venosus atrial septal defects (ASDs) and patent foramen ovale. The management of ostium primum and sinus venosus defects is by surgery because of associated abnormalities, namely, cleft in the mitral valve causing mitral regurgitation in ostium primum defects and partial anomalous pulmonary venous connection in sinus venosus defects and is addressed in Chapter 1. Patent foramen ovale (PFO) in relation to presumed paradoxical embolism, platypnea-orthodeoxia syndrome, migraine, decompression illness and others may also require closure and the considerations for closure of such PFOs are different than those of closure of ostium secundum ASDs and some of these are discussed in other chapters in this book and will not be addressed in this chapter. In this chapter only ostium secundum ASDs in adult subjects will be discussed; I will address issues related to why, when and how should atrial septal defects be closed in these subjects. The methods of transcatheter closure in adults will also be reviewed as are the approaches to occlude complex forms of ASD.

2. Why should atrial septal defects be closed in adults?

In the past it was generally thought that closure ASDs in adult subjects is not necessary if they are not symptomatic. Some early studies (Ward 1994, Gatzoulis et al 1996, Webb 2001) suggested that there is no major benefit if surgical closure is performed in adulthood. Based on more recent analysis however, it would appear that the ASDs should be closed as and when they are identified. The purpose of this section of this chapter is to present evidence that the ASDs in adults should be closed.

2.1 Evidence in favor of closing ASDs in adults

In this section I will review some of the published evidence supporting closure of ASDs in all adults

2.1.1 Complications in unrepaired ASD patients

In a follow-up study (Rosas et al 2004) of 200 patients older than 40 years (49 ± 9 years) with unrepaired ASD for 2 to 22 years, it was found that 37 (18.5%) had major events, namely heart failure in seven, sudden death in five, severe pulmonary infection in 13, embolism in five, stroke in four and miscellaneous complications in three. In addition, more than half of the patients had dyspnea at follow-up evaluation. Predictors of complications were analyzed and age at presentation, elevated pulmonary artery pressures and O2 saturation less than 80% were found to be associated with complications. These data suggest that major cardiovascular events are likely to occur in older adult patients with unrepaired ASD.

2.1.2 Safety and efficacy of surgical closure

Horvath et al (1991) examined safety and efficacy of surgical closure of ASDs. In this study, surgical closure was performed in 166 patients with a mean age of 44 years who had an average pulmonary to systemic flow ratio (Qp:Qs) of 3.0:1.0. The operative mortality was 1.2% (two deaths). The remaining patients were followed for a mean of 7.5 years. The overall survival and event-free survival rates were 98% and 97% at five years, respectively. Similarly, ten-year overall (94%) and event-free (92%) survival rates were high. Their (Horvath et al 1991) conclusion was that surgical closure is safe and effective with high event-free survival rates.

Konstantinides et al (1995) made a comparison of surgical closure with medical follow-up without surgery. One hundred-seventy-nine patients older than 40 years were examined; 84 of these had surgical closure while 95 had no surgery. The follow-up duration for both groups was 10 years. The actuarial 10-Year survival rate was 95% for the surgery group and 84% for no surgery group. In addition surgery also appears to have prevented deterioration of NYHA functional class. Based on these data the authors (Konstantinides et al 1995) conclude that surgical repair of ASD in adult subjects increases long-term survival and decreases functional deterioration when compared to medical therapy (no surgery).

2.1.3 Effect of ASD closure on cardiac function

Myocardial performance index (MPI), a Doppler-derived non-geometric measure of ventricular function, has been used to for quantitative assessment of ventricular function in patients with congenital heart disease both in adults and children; this measure appears to be relatively independent of changes in preload and afterload (Eidem 2000). Right ventricular (RV) MPI did not improve following surgical closure of ASD despite relief of RV volume overload (Eidem 2000). This was attributed to adverse effect of cardiopulmonary bypass on ventricular function. Salehian et al (2005) evaluated twenty-five patients at a mean age 46 years prior to and 3 months (mean) after device closure of ASD. Right ventricular MPI improved from 0.35 ± 0.14 to 0.28 ± 0.09 ($p = 0.004$) while left ventricular MPI enhanced from 0.37 ± 0.12 to 0.31 ± 0.11 ($p = 0.04$) (Figure 1). These authors (Salehian et al 2005) conclude that ASD closure improves cardiac function.

2.1.4 Effect of ASD closure on functional capacity

Improvement in functional capacity following ASD closure was studied by Brochu et al (2002). Thirty-seven patients with a mean age of 49 years whose mean Qp:Qs was 2:1 were evaluated. The VO2 max was measured and NYHA classification assessed prior to and 6 months after ASD closure. They found that VO2 max improved from 23 ± 6 to 27 ± 7 ($p < 0.0001$) following ASD closure. Fifteen out of 37 patients were in NYHA Class I prior to

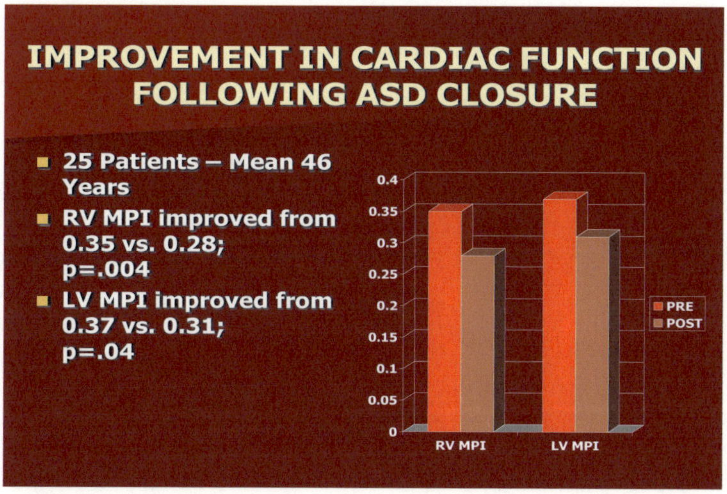

Fig. 1. Bar diagram demonstrating improvement in right ventricular (RV) and left ventricular (LV) myocardial performance index (MPI) following closure of atrial septal defect (ASD). PRE, before atrial septal defect closure; POST, three months after closure (constructed from the data of Salehian et al 2005).

surgery whereas 35 out of 37 patients were in NYHA Class I ($p < 0.0001$) six months after surgical closure. Thus, these authors' data demonstrated improvement in functional capacity following ASD closure (Brochu et al 2002).

2.2 Summary of why should atrial septal defects should be closed in adults

Based on review of the above and other reports, I conclude that untreated ASD patients tend to have decreased event-free survival rates when compared to normal population and surgical closure is safe and effective with high event-free survival rates. ASD closure also prevents functional deterioration, improves cardiac function and increases functional capacity. Consequently all adult patients with ASD should undergo closure of ASD.

3. When should atrial septal defects be closed in adults?

Murphy et al (1990) examined the effect of age at surgical closure of ASD. Patients who had surgical closure of ASD, performed between 1956 and 1960 at Mayo Clinic, were studied; they followed 123 patients and compared their actuarial survival rates with those of normal population. In the groups of patients who had surgery after 24 years of age, the actuarial survival rates are lower (Figure 2). When surgery is performed prior to 24 years of age, there was no significant difference in survival rates. The earlier the surgery was performed the better were the 27-year survival rates (Figure 2).

Based on these data Murphy concludes that early intervention may be beneficial; earlier the closure, the better is the long-term outlook. Consequently, it is prudent to close hemodynamically significant ASDs in all adults. Since there is no advantage in waiting beyond 24 years of age, the closure should be performed at the time of identification of the case.

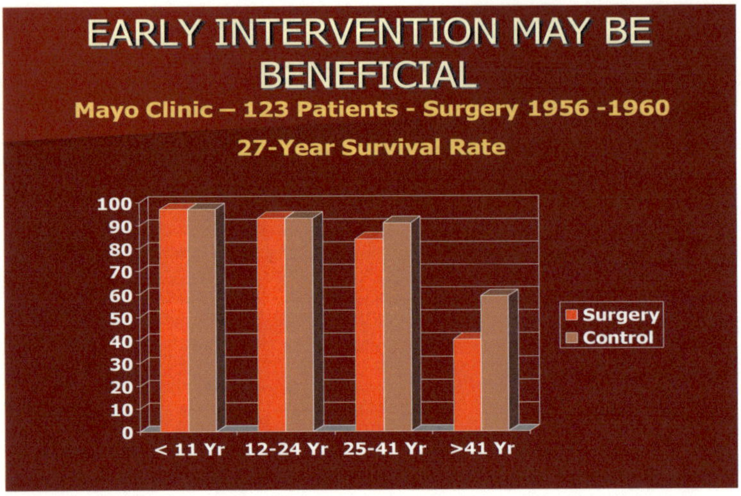

Fig. 2. Bar diagram (constructed from the data of Murphy et al 1990) depicting 27-year survival rates following closure of atrial septal defect by surgery; these data were compared with those of normal population. If surgery is performed prior to 24 years of age, there was no significant difference in survival rates. However, the survival rates are lower when surgical closure is performed later.

4. How should atrial septal defects be closed in adults

Following the introduction of cardiopulmonary bypass techniques for open heart surgery and the description of surgical closure of atrial septal defect (ASD) by Gibbon, Lillehei and Kirklin in 1950s, it rapidly became a standard form of treatment for atrial defects. The conventional treatment of choice of moderate and large defects until recently is surgical correction. Although surgical closure of ASDs is safe and effective with low mortality (Galal et al 1994, Pastorek et al 1994), the morbidity associated with sternotomy/thoracotomy is unavoidable. Consequently, substantial efforts have been made by the cardiology community to develop a non-surgical, catheter-based method of ASD occlusion. Since the initial description in mid 1970s by King & Mills and their associates (King and Mills 1974, Mills and King 1976, King et al 1976) of an atrial septal defect occluding device, a number of other devices, reviewed elsewhere (Chopra and Rao 2001, Rao 2003c) and in Chapter 1 of this book, were developed. However, Amplatzer Septal Occluder and HELEX are the only two devices approved for general clinical use by the US Food and Drug Administration (FDA) at the present time. Consequently, two methods of ASD closure, namely, surgical and transcatheter are now available.

4.1 Surgical vs. transcatheter closure

Studies, though limited in number, comparing surgical with device closure suggest similar effectiveness (Berger et al 1999, Du et al 2002, Durongpisitkul 2002, Bialkowski 2004). However, the device closure is less invasive, requires no cardio-pulmonary bypass. The device closure also appears to have less number of complications (10% vs. 31%), require less hospital stay (1 day vs. 4.3 days), and is less expensive (US $ 11,000 vs. $ 21,000) (Kim and Hijazi, 2002). The device closure techniques proved to be safe, cost-effective and favorably compare with surgical closure (Berger et al 1999, Du et al 2002, Kim and Hijazi 2002, Durongpisitkul 2002, Bettencourt et al 2003, Bialkowski 2004). Transcatheter occlusion of ASDs using various devices (Rao 2003a) is now an established practice in most centers providing state of the art care to patients with heart disease.

4.2 Surgical closure

When surgical closure is contemplated, a median sternotomy or a right sub mammary incision is made under general anesthesia. The aorta and vena cavae are cannulated and the patient is placed on cardiopulmonary bypass and right atriatomy is performed. The defect is exposed and closed either by approximating the defect margins with suture material or by using a pericardial patch, depending upon the size of the defect.

However, at the present time, surgical repair is largely reserved for ASDs with poor septal rims in which the interventional cardiologist opines that defect is difficult to close with trans-catheter methodology or was unsuccessful in closing the defect. If intra-cardiac repair of other defects is contemplated, surgical closure of ASD could also be performed at the same time.

4.3 Transcatheter closure

A number of devices are available to the interventional cardiologist for closure of ASD, but selection of an appropriate device is difficult because of lack of randomized clinical trials. Some studies (Formigari et al 1998, Walsh et al 1999, Sievert et al 1999, Keppeir 1999, Godart et al 2000, Butera et al 2004) compared the results of two or more devices, as and when the new deices became available. But, these studies are neither randomized nor blinded in their design and are unlikely to shed any more light than feasibility, safety and effectiveness studies of single devices. Given the current economical, ethical and medical considerations, a prospective randomized clinical trial utilizing all the eligible devices may not be possible. Therefore, selection of the device has largely been based on results of clinical trials conducted separately by the inventor or manufacturer of the device. I have carefully compared (Rao 1998a, Rao 1998b, Rao 2000, Rao 2003c) the implantation feasibility (ratio of implantations vs. patients taken to the catheterization laboratory with the intent to occlude), percentage of device dislodgements/miss-placements/embolizations, percent of patients with effective occlusion and re-intervention-free rates during follow-up; these results were tabulated elsewhere (Rao 2000, Rao 2003c). These comparisons revealed that these parameters are similar and comparable for most, if not all devices that I had the opportunity to evaluate. While the feasibility, safety and effectiveness are most important, availability, cost, size of the delivery sheath and other factors should also be considered in the process of device selection.

Of the devices tabulated in the prior publications (Rao 2000, Rao 2003c) and others that entered clinical trials since those reviews (see chapter 1), some devices were discontinued, shelved or withdrawn because of different reasons and some others continue to be in clinical trials either within or outside the US. Amplatzer (AGA Medical Corp., Golden Valley, MN) and HELEX (W.L. Gore, Flagstaff, AZ) devices are the only devices approved by the FDA at the present time, for general clinical use for closure of the ASDs.

The Amplatzer septal occluder is the most commonly used ASD closure device worldwide at the present time. The feasibility, safety and efficacy of device occlusion are based on self-expandable, retrievable and re-positionable design of the device (Hamdan et al 2003). Even very large defects can be closed successfully with Amplatzer device using a variety of techniques (Nagm and Rao 2004, Rao 2007).

4.3.1 Protocol for ASD closure

4.3.1.1 Diagnosis and indications

After a clinical and echocardiographic diagnosis of moderate to large ostium secundum ASD is made, consideration for transcatheter closure should be given. Because of poor echo windows, most adult subjects require transesophageal echocardiography (TEE) to confirm the diagnosis, to quantify its size and define the septal rims. The indications for closure in adults are similar to those used in children (see Chapter 1) and are echocardiographic finding of right ventricular volume overloading and/or catheterization findings of Qp:Qs greater than 1.5:1.0. The reasons for closure of ASDs in children are prevention of pulmonary vascular obstructive disease in adulthood, to prevent arrhythmias and to prevent symptoms later in life. Additional reasons in adult subjects are to prevent heart failure, prevent functional deterioration, improve myocardial function and prevent paradoxical embolism.

4.3.1.2 Consent, catheterization and transesophageal or intracardiac echocardiography

Informed consent is obtained and cardiac catheterization is performed preparatory to transcatheter occlusion, at the same sitting. Right heart catheterization is undertaken percutaneously to confirm the clinical and echocardiographic diagnosis with particular attention to exclude partial anomalous pulmonary venous return. Some interventionalists perform left atrial cineangiogram in a left axial oblique view (30^0 LAO and 30^0 Cranial) with the catheter positioned in the right upper pulmonary vein at its junction with the left atrium while others do not routinely perform this angiogram. Transesophageal (TEE) or intracardiac (ICE) (Hijazi et al 2001) echocardiography to measure the size of the ASD, to visualize entry of all pulmonary veins into the left atrium and to examine the atrial septal rims is then undertaken.

4.3.1.3 Device description and implantation

Detailed descriptions of Amplatzer Septal Occluder and HELEX devices and their implantation were included in Chapter 1 of this book. Device placement protocol in adults is similar to that described for children and will not be detailed here except to state that the procedure is performed more often under ICE guidance in adults than in children and Clopidogrel 75 mg/day for the first 2 to 3 months after device implantation in addition to Aspirin 185 or 325 mg/Kg/day by mouth for six months is given in adults. However, discussion of some issues germane to adult subjects and device closure of complex ASDs will be included hereunder.

4.3.1.4 Precautions in elderly subjects prior to ASD closure

Reduced diastolic elasticity of the left ventricle is particularly seen in the elderly, causing restrictive filling of the left ventricle (Holzer et al 2005, Al-Hindi et al 2009). The ASD decompresses the left atrium and prevents high left ventricular end-diastolic pressure. The pop-off mechanism no longer exists after the ASD is closed. Consequently, the patients may develop pulmonary edema and may require prolonged mechanical ventilation and inotropic support (Al-Hindi et al 2009). If the left atrial pressure is higher than 15 mmHg, temporary balloon occlusion of the defect for 10 to 15 minutes and re-measuring the left atrial pressure (or pulmonary artery wedge pressure) is recommended. If the pressure increases by more than 5 mmHg, the defect should not be closed at that sitting. But the patient should be treated with afterload reducing agents and diuretics for one to two weeks. The patient should be restudied following afore-mentioned treatment, measuring the left atrial pressures during balloon occlusion of the ASD. If the pressure does not increase by more than 5 mmHg, device occlusion of ASD may be undertaken. If the pressure continues to be high, a fenestrated device may have to be used (Peters et al 2006, Kretschmar et al 2010, MacDonald et al 2011, Kenny 2011).

4.3.1.5 Precautions in subjects with pulmonary hypertension

In some adult ASD patients pulmonary hypertension may be present. In these patients, a particular attention should be paid to calculate pulmonary vascular resistance. Pulmonary vascular resistance (PVR) may be calculated:

PVR = (Mean PA presence - Mean LA pressure)/Pulmonary blood flow index

Where, PA and LA are pulmonary artery and left atrium respectively.

The calculated resistance is normally between 1 and 2 units and a resistance higher than 3.0 units is considered elevated. Marked elevation of the resistance (>8.0 units) contraindicates closure of the ASD. When the resistance is elevated, oxygen and other vasodilating agents, particularly Nitric oxide (NO) should be administered to demonstrate the reversibility. In addition, pulmonary arterial wedge angiography and sometimes, even lung biopsy may be necessary to determine the suitability for closure. Patients with calculated pulmonary vascular resistance less than 8 wood units with a Qp:Qs >1.5 are generally considered suitable candidates for ASD occlusion. In patients with increased pulmonary vascular resistance, if the calculated resistance drops to levels below 8 units after administering oxygen or other vasodilator agents (NO), the patient becomes a candidate for closure of ASD.

If the results of the testing of pulmonary vascular reactivity are marginal or the pulmonary vascular resistance remains elevated (>8.0 units) following vasodilator testing, a fenestrated Amplatzer device may be implanted across the ASD (Lammerset al 2007, Kretschmar et al 2010). The device will reduce the left-to-right shunt, thus removing the effect of continued increase in pulmonary blood flow and may result in improvement. Should the pulmonary vascular resistance continue to increase despite the fenestrated device closure, the fenestrations in the device will serve as a pop-off escape mechanism and maintain near normal cardiac index, though at the expense of arterial oxygen desaturation.

4.3.2 Approaches for closure of complex ASDs

Secundum ASDs located centrally in the atrial septum are found in only 24% of cases (Podnar et al 2001). These authors reviewed the characteristic of ASDs in 190 patients who had transcatheter or surgical repair and found deficient superior anterior rim in 42%, deficient inferior posterior rim in 10%, perforated aneurysm of the atrial septum in 8%, multiple defects in 7%, deficient inferior anterior and superior anterior rims in 3%, deficient inferior posterior and posterior rims in 2% and deficient inferior anterior, superior posterior and coronary sinus rims in 1 % each. In another study complex ASDs were present in 40 (28%) of 143 patients (Pedra et al 2004). These authors arbitrarily defined complex anatomy as ASDs with stretched diameters larger than 26 mm with a deficient (<4 mm) rim in 23 (16%), two separate defects with a distance greater than 7 mm in 8 (5.6%), fenestrated atrial septum in 5 (3.5%) or redundant and hyper mobile (>10 mm) atrial septum in 4 (2.8%). In the ensuing paragraphs I will address how the complex ASDs can be closed by transcatheter methodology.

4.3.2.1 Large defects with deficient anterior-superior rim

Pedra et al (2004) defined large ASD as a defect with a stretched diameter > 26 mm. Similar definitions were used by most other cardiologists. While it goes without saying that large defects need large devices to close, the interventionalist needs to consider whether the left atrium could accommodate a large device and whether such a large device would interfere with atrio-ventricular valve function or obstruct vena caval or pulmonary venous blood return. Deficient anterosuperior rim is frequently encountered with large ASDs and indeed, in my own personal experience most patients I attempted to occlude with various devices were found to have deficient anterior superior rim. Other cardiologists (Podnar et al 2001, Berger et al 2001, Chessa et al 2002, Mathewson et al 2004) had similar experiences. With deficient anterosuperiorr rim, the disks of the Amplatzer straddle the ascending aorta. With other double disk devices the left atrial disk sits on the back of aorta.

4.3.2.1.1 Amplatzer device

While deploying the Amplatzer device in ASDs with deficient anterior superior rim, the left atrial disk tends to become perpendicular to the atrial septum leading to prolapse of the left disk into the right atrium. Several techniques have been proposed to overcome such difficulties; these were reviewed elsewhere (Nagm and Rao 2004, Rao 2007). The left atrial disk of the device is deployed in the right upper or left upper pulmonary vein and the waist and the right atrial disk are released while simultaneously withdrawing the deployed left atrial disk against the atrial septum; this technique has been successfully used by several investigators (Berger et al 2001, Du et al 2002, Chessa et al 2002, Harper et al 2002, Varma et al 2004, Fu et al 2007). While the device placement may be successful with these techniques, there is some concern regarding the risk of injury to the pulmonary vein. Heat-bending the distal portion of the delivery sheath 360 degrees along with cutting off the tip of the sheath ≥ 45 degrees toward its inner circumference is another technique used to help overcome the prolapse of the left disk into the right atrium (Cooke et al 2001, Mathewson et al 2004, Varma et al 2004). Hausdorf sheath (Cook, Bloomington, IN), a specially designed sheath with two curves at the end may help align the left atrial disk parallel to the septum and this delivery catheter has successfully been used by some workers (Staniloae et al 2003, Pedra et al 2004, Varma et al 2004). Holding the left atrial disk with the tip of a reinforced dilator (Abdul Wahab 2003), sizing balloon catheter (Dalvi et al 2005, Flores et al 2008) or a steerable guide catheter (Nounou et al 2008) to prevent its prolapse into the right atrium has also been employed successfully. Kutty et al (2007) cut the sheath to create a straight catheter with a side-hole, the so called SSH modification and were successful in positioning the device in 120 of 122 (98.4%) patients; this is in contradistinction to the successful deployment of the device in 14 of 18 (78%) patients with the use of standard Amplatzer delivery sheath. The cardiologists should consider all options reviewed above and select the method that is most likely to result in successful implantation of the device in their patient.

4.3.2.1.2 HELEX device

Since the HELEX device is not suitable for large defects, it should not be used to occlude large ASDs.

4.3.2.2 Large defects with deficient postero-inferior rim

Some of the large ASDs are associated with deficient posterior-inferior (PI) rim (Pedra et al 2004) making the device implantation difficult. Varma et al (2004) studied reasons for unsuccessful Amplatzer implantations and found deficient inferior rim as an explanation for unsuccessful deployments. Closure of a large ASD with deficient or absent PI rim is a real challenge. Insufficient number of cases with deficient PI rim reported in most series makes it even more difficult to have a consensus. Du et al (2002) reported 23 patients with deficient rims; of these 3 patients had deficient inferior or posterior rims. Two patients had 2 mm of posterior rim and the third had a 4 mm posterior rim. These 3 patients' ASDs were successfully closed. Mathewson et al (2004) defined absent PI rim as a rim < 3 mm. As the difference in radius length between right and left atrial disks of the Amplatzer device is 2-3 mm, a rim < 3 mm will not allow both disks to hang on both sides of the rim. They found that defects with absent PI rim tend to be larger in diameter. They concluded that, although a stable Amplatzer device deployment is possible, these defects are more liable for complications such as pulmonary vein or inferior vena caval obstruction, encroachment onto the anterior mitral leaflet or frank embolization (Mathewson et al 2004). The number of cases reported is too small to make a generalized conclusion as to what is the best approach to address these ASDs.

4.3.2.3 Multiple or fenestrated defects

Multiple or fenestrated ASDs may be successfully occluded by different techniques or devices. One method used for addressing fenestrated defects was to perform balloon atrial septostomy to create a single large defect which was then closed with a single large Amplatzer device (Carano et al 2001). While these authors were successful in occluding the defect, I am not in favor of using such a technique. A large single Amplatzer device may be deployed in the larger defect to occlude two or more smaller defects as used by Szkutnik et al (2004) and others (Roman et al 2002). While examining this technique, Szkutnik et al (2004) found that a smaller defect less than 7 mm distance from the larger defect had a 100% closure rate at 1 month follow-up. The device in the larger defect decreases the distance between the two defects or even compress the smaller defect (Szkutnik et al 2004). However, if the distance between the two defects is >7 mm, a residual left to right shunt persisted (Szkutnik et al 2004). Several investigators (Pedra et al 1998, Bandel et al 2002, Roman et al 2002, Pinto and Dalvi 2005, Awad et al 2007, Tillman et al 2008, Butera et al 2010, Duygu et al 2010. Cho et al 2011) used two Amplatzer devices to close two ASDs concurrently. Extremely rarely three devices (Lander et al 2004, Arcidiacono et al 2008) may be required to completely close all the defects. Multiple defects may also be closed with a large single device such as CardioSeal device (Pedra et al 2000, Evert et al 2001) or Cribriform Amplatzer device (Hijazi et al 2003, Numan et al 2008).

While the conventional method of imaging the atrial septum and monitoring device deployment is two-dimensional TEE or ICE, more recently three-dimensional transthoracic (Arcidiacono et al 2008) or transesophageal (Kuo et al 2011) echocardiography has been used. However, it is not clear whether three dimensional imaging techniques are superior to two dimensional techniques.

Based on these observations and other reports as well as our personal experience, the following recommendations may be made. If the smaller defect is hemodynamically significant, but is far (>7 mm) from the larger defect, two devices should be used. After verifying good position of both devices, release of smaller device should precede the release of larger device. Extremely rarely three devices (Lander et al 2004, Arcidiacono et al 2008) may be needed to completely close all the defects. If the defects are close to each other (<7mm) Cribriform Amplatzer device (Hijazi et al 2003, Zanchetta et al 2005, Numan et al 2008), large enough to cover all the defects may be used. We used both these techniques with good success.

4.3.2.4 Anuerysmal atrial septum

Single or multiple defects with septal aneurysm represent a different type of complex ASD. Such defects may be better dealt with devices that don't rely on stenting the defect (for example Amplatzer device) in order to achieve stabilization in the septum. Devices with two discs such as the hybrid buttoned device (Rao 2003d), the HELEX, the CardioSeal or the Cribriform Amplatzer (Musto et al 2009) are more appropriate choices to close such defects. Closing two small but distant defects within an aneurismal atrial septum may effectively close both defects but carry a higher risk of later development of thrombus formation (Krumsdorf et al 2004). We have successfully closed defects associated with atrial septal aneurysms with hybrid buttoned devices (Figure 3) by compressing the aneurysm between the occluder and the square shaped counter-occluder (Rao 2003d).

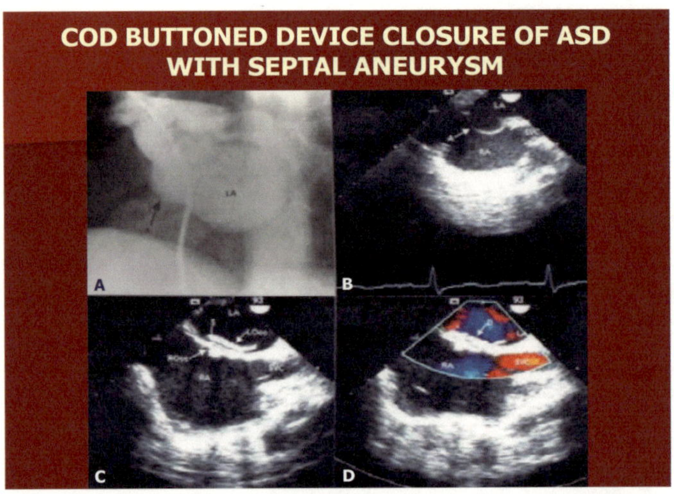

Fig. 3. Selected left atrial (LA) cineangiographic (A) and transesophageal echocardiographic (B) frames showing atrial septal aneurysm (A, arrow). After closure of the atrial septal defect with a hybrid buttoned device (C), the aneurysm is sandwiched between the left atrial (LA) component of the device (LOcc) and right atrial (RA) component of the device (ROcc). No residual shunt is seen (D). The superior vena cava (SVC) is unobstructed.

4.3.3 Conclusions – Approaches for closure of complex ASDs

It may be concluded that most complex ASDs can be closed successfully either by using traditional or special devices or techniques. Defects with deficient or absent PI rim continue to be challenging for most interventionalists and may require surgical closure.

4.3.4 Long-term complications of transcatheter closure

Reports of erosion of the aortic wall by the Amplatzer device with development of aorta-to-right atrium (Chun 2003) or aorta-to-left atrium (Aggoun et al 2002) fistulae led to the suggestion of over-sizing the device (4 mm larger than the measured stretched diameter) in large defects with deficient anterior superior rim. This is meant to ensure that the device disks straddle and remain flared around the ascending aorta to prevent discrete areas of pressure where erosion may occur. Of course, when over-sizing the device, care must be taken not to interfere with atrio-ventricular valve function and venous return. Device migration and erosion of aorta (Amin et al 2004, AGA 2006) was observed during follow-up in 37 out of 35,000 (0.11% or 1 in 1,000) Amplatzer device implants world-wide. This complication was also similar in the US study population: 18 out of 15,900 implants (0.12% or 1 in 1,000). Review of data by the Review Board and AGA Medical (AGA 2006) suggested that the device erosion is related to over-sizing of the device (Figure 4) and recommended that device size >1.5 times the TEE/ICE diameter of ASD should not be used.

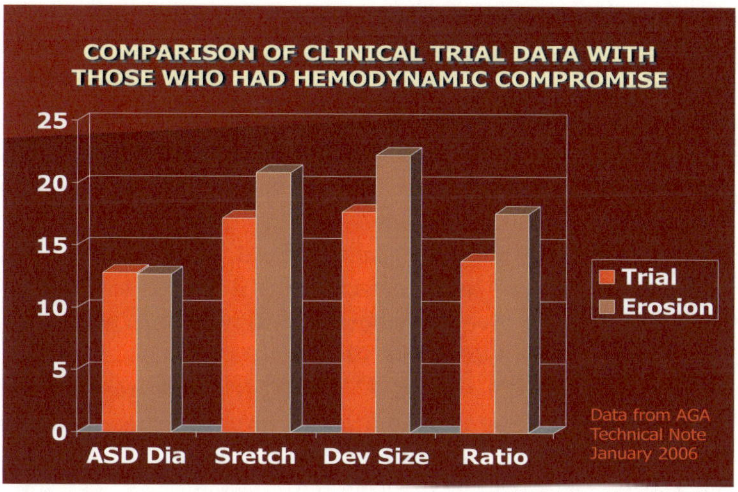

Fig. 4. Bar diagram demonstrating relationship of atrial septal defect (ASD) and device size data between the group of patients without perforation (Trial) and those that had perforation (Erosion). The diameter (Dia) of the ASD was similar in both groups whereas the stretched diameter (Stretch), device size (Dev size) and ratio of device to ASD (Ratio) were larger in the patients who had perforation than those who did not. Based on these data a recommendation made not to use devices larger 1.5 X ASD size (Constructed from the data of AGA 2006).

5. Summary and conclusions

ASDs in adult subjects should be closed at presentation, electively, irrespective of their age. Evidence was presented to indicate that hemodynamically significant (right ventricular volume overload) ASDs in adults should be transcatheter occluded irrespective of symptomatology. While surgical closure is safe and effective, device closure carries less morbidity. Multiple devices have been investigated over the last few decades, but only Amplatzer and HELEX devices received FDA approval as of this time. The Amplatzer is useful in most ASDs while the HELEX device is useful in small and medium-sized defects. Some procedural details were mentioned with particular emphasis on the need for test occlusion of ASD in the elderly. Approaches taken to occlude ASDs with complex anatomy were also reviewed. Amplatzer device appears to be best available option at the present time. Careful attention to the details of the technique are mandatory to achieve a successful outcome

6. References

[1] Abdul Wahab, H.; Bairam, AR.; Cao, Q,; Hijazi, ZM. (2003) Novel technique to prevent prolapse of the Amplatzer septal occluder through large atrial septal defect. *Cathet Cardiovascu Intervent,* Vol. 60, No. 4, pp. 543-545.

[2] AGA Medical Technical Note, January 2006:1-4.

[3] Aggoun, Y.; Gallet, B.; Acar, P.; et al. (2002) Perforation of the aorta after percutaneous closure of an atrial septal defect with an Amplatzer prosthesis with acute severe hemolysis. *Arch Mal Coeur Vaiss,* Vol. 95, No. 5, pp. 479-482.

[4] Al-Hindi, A.; Cao, QL.; Hijazi, ZM. (2009) Transcatheter closure of secundum atrial septal defect in the elderly. *J Invasive Cardiol* , Vol. 21, No. 2, pp. 70-75.

[5] Amin, Z.; Hijazi, ZM.; Bass, JL.; et al. (2004) Erosion of Amplatzer septal occluder device after closure of secundum atrial septal defect: Review of registry of complications and recommendations to minimize future risk. *Cathet Cardiovascu Intervent,* Vol. 63, No. 4, pp. 491-502.

[6] Arcidiacon, C.; Gaio, G.; Butera, G.; Carminati, M. (2008) Percutaneous closure of multiple secundum atrial septal defects using 3 Amplatzer atrial septal occluder devices: evaluation by live transthoracic 3-dimensional echocardiography. *Circ Cardiovasc Imaging,* Vol. 1, No. 2, pp. c15-16.

[7] Awad, SM.; Garay, FF.; Cao, QL.; Hijazi, ZM. (2007) Multiple Amplatzer septal occluder devices for multiple atrial communications: immediate and long-term follow-up results. *Catheter Cardiovasc Interv, Vol.* 70, No. 2, pp. 265-273.

[8] Bandel, JW.; Collet, HC.; Patiño, J. (2002) The versatility of the Amplatzer Septal Occluder for the management of multiple atrial septal defects in a patient with dextrocardia and situs inversus. *J Invasive Cardiol,* Vol. 14, No. 6, pp. 340-342.

[9] Berger, F.; Ewert, P.; Abdul-Khalid, H.; et al. (2001) Percutaneous closure of large atrial septal defects with the Amplatzer septal occluder: technical overkill or recommendable alternative treatment. *J Intervent Cardiol,* Vol. 14, No. 1, pp. 63-67.

[10] Berger, F.; Vogel, M.; Alexi-Meskishvili, V.; Lange, PE. (1999) Comparison of results and complications of surgical and Amplatzer device closure of atrial septal defects. *J Thorac Cardiovasc Surg,* Vol. 118, No. 4, pp. 674-678.

[11] Bettencourt, N.; Salome, N.; Carneiro, F.; et al. (2003) Atrial septal closure in adults : surgery versus Amplatzer—comparison of results. *Rev Port Cardiol,* Vol. 22, No. 10, pp. 1203-1211.

[12] Bialkowski, J.; Karwot, B.; Szkutnik, M.; et al. (2004) Closure of atrial septal defects in children: surgery versus Amplatzer device implantation. *Tex Heart Inst J,* Vol. 31, No. 3, pp. 220-223.

[13] Brochu, MC.; Baril, JF.; Dore, A.; et al. (2002) Improvement in exercise capacity in asymptomatic and mildly symptomatic adults after atrial septal defect percutaneous closure. *Circulation,* Vol. 106, No. 14, pp. 1821-1826.

[14] Butera, G.; Carminati, M.; Chessa, M.; et al. (2004) CardioSEAL/STARflex versus Amplatzer devices for percutaneous closure of small to moderate (up to 18 mm) atrial septal defects. *Am Heart J,* Vol. 148, No. 3, pp. 507-510.

[15] Butera, G.; Romagnoli, E.; Saliba, Z.; et al. (2010) Percutaneous closure of multiple defects of the atrial septum: procedural results and long-term follow-up. *Catheter Cardiovasc Interv,* Vol. 76, No. 1, pp. 121-128.

[16] Carano, N.; Hagler, DJ.; Agnetti, A.; Squarcia, U. (2001) Device closure of fenestrated atrial septal defect: use of a single Amplatz atrial occluder after balloon atrial septostomy to create a single defect. *Catheter Catrdiovsc Interentv,* Vol. 53, No. 2, pp. 203-207.

[17] Chessa, M.; Carminati, M.; Buetera, G.; et al. (2002) Early and late complications associated with transcatheter occlusion of secundum atrial septal defect. *J Am Coll Cardiol,* Vol. 39, No. 2, pp. 1061-1065.

[18] Cho, MJ.; Song, J.; Kim, SJ.; et al. (2011) Transcatheter closure of multiple atrial septal defects with the Amplatzer device. *Korean Circ J,* Vol. 41, No. 9, pp. 549-51. Epub 2011 Sep 29.

[19] Chopra, PS.; Rao, PS. (2000) History of the Development of Atrial Septal Occlusion Devices. Current Intervent Cardiol Reports, Vol. 2, No. 1, 63-69.

[20] Chun, DS.; Turrentine, MW.; Moustapha, A.; Hoyer MH. (2003) Development of aorta-to-right atrial fistula following closure of secundum atrial septal defect using the Amplatzer septal occluder. *Catheter Cardiovasc Intervent,* Vol. 58, No. 2, pp. 246-251.

[21] Cooke, JC.; Gelman, JS.; Harper, RW. (2001) Echocardiographic role in the deployment of the Amplatzer septal occluder device in adults. *J Am Society of Echocardiogr,* Vol. 14, No. 6, pp. 588-594.

[22] Dalvi, BV.; Pinto, RJ.; Gupta, A. (2005) New technique for device closure of large atrial septal defects. *Cathet Cardiovascu Interv,* Vol. 64, No. 1, 102-107.

[23] Du, ZD.; Hijazi, ZM.; Kleinman, CS.; et al. (2002) Comparison between transcatheter and surgical closure of secundum atrial septal defect in children and adults: results of multicenter nonrandomized trial. *J Am Coll Cardiol,* Vol. 39, No. 11, pp. 1836-1844.

[24] Durongpisitkul, K.; Soongswang, J.; Laohaprasitiporn, D.; et al. (2002) Comparison of atrial septal defect closure using amplatzer septal occluder with surgery. *Pediatr Cardiol,* Vol. 23, No. 1, pp. 36-40.

[25] Duygu, H.; Acet, H.; Kocabas, U.; et al. (2010) Percutaneous successful closure of dual atrial septal defect with two Amplatzer septal occluder devices. *Clin Res Cardiol,* Vol. 99, No. 5, pp. 29-31.

[26] Eidem, BW.; O'Leary, PW.; Tei, C.; Seward, JB. (2000)Usefulness of the myocardial performance index for assessing right ventricular function in congenital heart disease. *Am J Cardiol,* Vol. 86, No. 6, pp. 654-658.

[27] Ewert, P.; Berger, F.; Kretschmar O, et al. (2001) Feasibility of transcatheter closure of multiple defects within the oval fossa. *Cardiol Young,* Vol. 11, No. 3, pp. 314 -319.

[28] Flores, RA.; Salgado, A.; Antúnez, SP.; et al. (2008) Correction of the perpendicular positioning of the Amplatzer device during closure of an ostium secundum atrial septal defect. *Rev Esp Cardiol,* Vol. 61, No. 7, pp. 714-718.

[29] Formigari, R.; Santoro, G.; Rosetti, L.; et al. (1998) Comparison of three different atrial septal defect occluding devices. *Am J Cardiol,* Vol. 82, No. 5, pp. 690-692.

[30] Fu, YC.; Cao, QL.; Hijazi, ZM. (2007) Device closure of large atrial septal defects: technical considerations. *J Cardiovasc Med (Hagerstown),* Vol. 8, No. 1, pp. 30-33.

[31] Galal, MO.; Wobst, A.; Halees, Z.; et al. (1994) Perioperative complications following surgical closure of atrial septal defect type II in 232 patients - a baseline study. *Europ Heart J,* Vol. 15, No. 10, pp. 1381-1384.

[32] Gatzoulis, MA.; Redington, AN.; Somerville, J.; et al. (1996) Should atrial septal defects in adults be closed? *Ann Thorac Surg,* Vol. 61, No. 2, pp. 657–659.

[33] Godart, F.; Rey, C.; Francart, C.; et al. (2000) Experience in one centre using the buttoned device for occlusion of atrial septal defect: comparison with the Amplatzer septal occluder. *Cardiol Young,* Vol. 10, No. 5, pp. 527-533.

[34] Hamdan, MA.; Cao, Q.; Hijazi, ZM. (2003) Amplatzer septal occluder. In: *Catheter Based Devices for Treatment of Noncoronary Cardiovascular Disease in Adults and Children,* P.S. Rao, M.J. Kern. (Eds.): 51-59, Lippincott, Williams & Wilkins, Philadelphia, PA, USA.

[35] Harper, RW.; Mottram, PM.; McGaw, DJ. (2002) Closure of secundum atrial septal defects with the Amplatzer septal occluder device: techniques and problems. *Catheter Cardiovasc Intervent,* Vol. 57, No. 4, pp. 508-524.

[36] Hijazi, ZM.; and Cao, Q-L. (2003) Transcatheter closure of multi-fenestrated atrial septal defects using the new Amplatzer cribriform device. *Congental Cardiology Today,* Vol. 1, No. pp. 1-4.

[37] Hijazi, ZM., Wang, Z.; Cao, QL.; et al. (2001) Transcatheter closure of atrial septal defects and patent foramen ovale under intracardiac echocardiographic guidance: feasibility and comparison with transesophageal echocardiography. *Cath Cardiovasc Intervent,* Vol. 52, No. 2, pp. 194-199.

[38] Holzer, R.; Cao, QL.; Hijazi, ZM. (2005) Closure of a moderately large atrial septal defect with a self-fabricated fenestrated Amplatzer septal occluder in an 85-year-old patient with reduced diastolic elasticity of the left ventricle. *Catheter Cardiovasc Interv,* Vol. 64, No. 4, pp. 513-518

[39] Horvath, KA.; Burke, RP.; Collins, JJ. Jr.; Cohn, LH. (1991) Surgical treatment of adult atrial septal defect: early and long-term results. *J Am Coll Cardiol,* Vol. 20, No. 5, pp. 1156-1159.

[40] Kenny, D.; Cao, QL.; Hijazi, ZM. (2011) Fenestration of a Gore Helex Septal Occluder device in a patient with diastolic dysfunction of the left ventricle. *Catheter Cardiovasc Interv,* Vol. 78, No. 4, pp. 594-598

[41] Keppeir, P.; Rux, S.; Dirko, J.; et al. (1999) Transcatheter closure of 100 patent foramina ovalia in patients with unexplained stroke and suspected paradoxic embolism: a comparison of five different devices [abstract]. *Europ Heart J,* Vol. 20, No. 2, pp. 196.

[42] Kim, JJ.; Hijazi, ZM. (2002) Clinical outcomes and costs of Amplatzer transcatheter closure as compared with surgical closure of ostium secondum atrial septal defects. *Med Science Monitor,* Vol. 8, No. 12, pp. CR787-791.

[43] King, TD.; Mills NL. (1974) Nonoperative closure of atrial septal defects. *Surgery,* Vol. 75, No. 3, pp. 383-388.

[44] King, TD.; Thompson, SL.; Steiner, C.; et al. (1976) Secundum atrial septal defect: nonoperative closure during cardiac catheterization. *J Am Med Assoc,* Vol. 235, No. 23, pp. 2506-2509.

[45] Konstantinides, S.; Geibel, A.; Olschewski, M.; et al. (1995) A comparison of surgical and medical therapy for atrial septal defects in adults. *New Engl J Med,* Vol. 333, No. 8, pp. 469-473.

[46] Kretschmar, O.; Sglimbea, A.; Corti, R.; Knirsch, W. (2010) Shunt reduction with a fenestrated Amplatzer device. *Catheter Cardiovasc Interv,* Vol. 76, No. 4, pp. 564-571.

[47] Krumsdorf, U.; Ostermayer, S.; Ballinger, K.; et al. (2004) Incidence and clinical course of thrombus formation on atrial septal defect and patent foramen ovale closure devices in 1000 consecutive patients. *J Am Coll Cardiol,* Vol. 43, No. 2, 302-309.

[48] Kuo, BT.; Whitbeck, MG.; Gurley, JC.; Smith, MD. (2011) Double atrial septal defect: diagnosis and closure guidance with 3D transesophageal echocardiography. *Echocardiography,* Vol. 28, No. 6, pp. E115-117.

[49] Kutty, S.; Asnes, JD.; Srinath, G.; et al. (2007) Use of a straight, side-hole delivery sheath for improved delivery of Amplatzer ASD occluder. *Cathet Cardiovascular Interv,* Vol. 69, No. 1, pp. 15-20.

[50] Lammers, AE.; Derrick, G.; Haworth, SG.; et al. (2007) Efficacy and long-term patency of fenestrated Amplatzer devices in children. *Catheter Cardiovasc Interv,* Vol. 70, No. 4, pp. 578-584.

[51] Lander, SR.; Phillips, S.; Vallabhan, RC.; (2004) et al. Percutaneous closure of multiple atrial septal defects with three Amplatzer septal occluder devices. *Catheter Cardiovasc Interv,* Vol. 62, No. 4, pp. 526-529.

[52] Mathewson, JW.; Bichell, D.; Rothman, A.; Ing, FF. (2004) Absent posteroinferior and anterosuperior atrial septal defect rims: Factors affecting nonsurgical closure of large secundum defects using the Amplatzer occluder. *J Am Soc Echocardiogr,* Vol. 17, No. 1, pp. 62-69.

[53] MacDonald, ST.; Arcidiacono, C.; Butera, G. (2011) Fenestrated Amplatzer atrial septal defect occluder in an elderly patient with restrictive left ventricular physiology. *Heart,* Vol. 97, No.5, p. 438.

[54] Mills, NL.; King, TD. (1976) Nonoperative closure of left-to-right shunts. *J Thorac Cardiovasc Surg,* Vol. 72, No. 3, pp. 371-378.

[55] Murphy, JG.; Gersh, BJ.; McGoon, MD.; et al. (1990) Long-term outcome after surgical repair of isolated atrial septal defect. *New Engl J Med,* Vol. 323, No. 24, pp. 1645-1650.

[56] Musto, C.; Cifarelli, A.; Pandolfi, C.; et al. (2009) Transcatheter closure of patent foramen ovale associated with atrial septal aneurysm with Amplatzer Cribriform septal occluder. *J Invasive Cardiol,* Vol. 21, No. 6, pp. 290-293.

[57] Nagm, AM.; Rao, PS. (2004) Percutaneous occlusion of complex atrial septal defects (Editorial). *J Invasive Cardiol,* Vol. 16, No. 3, pp. 123-125.

[58] Nounou, M,; Harrison, A.; Kern, M. (2008) A novel technique using a steerable guide catheter to successfully deliver an Amplatzer septal occluder to close an atrial septal defect. *Catheter Cardiovasc Interv,* Vol. 72, No. 7, pp. 994-997.

[59] Numan, M.; El Sisi, A.; Tofeig, M.; et al. (2008) Cribriform amplatzer device closure of fenestrated atrial septal defects: feasibility and technical aspects. *Pediatr Cardiol,* Vol. 29, No. 3, pp. 530-535. Epub 2007 Nov 13.

[60] Pastorek, JS.; Allen, HD.; Davis, JT. (1994) Current outcomes of surgical closure of secundum atrial septal defect. Am J Cardiol, Vol. 74, No. 1, pp. 75-77.

[61] Pedra, CA.; Fontes-Pedra, SR.; Esteves, CA.; et al. (1998) Multiple atrial septal defects and patent ductus arteriosus: successful outcome using two Amplatzer septal occluders and Gianturco coils. *Cathet Cardiovasc Diagn,* Vol. 45, No. 3, pp. 257-259.

[62] Pedra, CA.; Pedra, SRF.; Esteves, CSA.; et al. (2004) Transcatheter closure of secundum atrial septal defects with complex anatomy. *J Invasive Cardiol,* Vol. 16, No. 3, pp. 117-122

[63] Pedra, CA.; Pihkala, J.; Lee, K-J.; et al. (2000) Transcatheter closure of atrial septal defects using the CardioSeal implant. *Heart,* Vol. 84, No. 3, pp. 320–326.

[64] Peters, B.; Ewert, P.; Schubert, S.; et al. (2006) Self-fabricated fenestrated Amplatzer occluders for transcatheter closure of atrial septal defect in patients with left ventricular restriction: midterm results. *Clin Res Cardiol,* Vol. 95, No. 2, pp. 88-92. Epub 2006 Jan 16.

[65] Pinto, RJ.; Dalvi, B. (2005) Closure of two atrial septal defects using two separate Amplatzer ASD devices. *Indian Heart J.* Vol. 57, No. 3, pp. 251-254.

[66] Podnar, T.; Martanovič, P.; Gavora, P.; Masura, J. (2001) Morphological variations of secundum - type atrial septal defects: Feasibility for percutaneous closure using Amplatzer septal occluders. *Catheter Cardiovasc Intervent,* Vol. 53, No. 3, pp. 386-391.

[67] Rao, PS. (1998a) Closure devices for atrial septal defect: which one to chose? (editorial). *Indian Heart J,* Vol. 50, No. 4, pp. 379-383.

[68] Rao, PS. (1998b) Transcatheter closure of atrial septal defects: Are we there yet? (editorial). *J Am Coll Cardiol,* Vol. 31, No. 5, pp. 1117-1119.

[69] Rao, PS. (2000) Summary and Comparison of Atrial Septal Defect Closure Devices. *Current Intervent Cardiol Reports,* Vol. 2, No. 4, pp. 367-376.

[70] Rao, PS. (2003a) Catheter Closure of Atrial Septal Defects (Editorial). *J Invasive Cardiol,* Vol. 15, No. pp. 398-400.

[71] Rao, PS. (2003b) History of atrial septal occlusion devices, In: *Catheter Based Devices for Treatment of Noncoronary Cardiovascular Disease in Adults and Children,* P.S. Rao, M.J. Kern. (Eds.): 1-9, Lippincott, Williams & Wilkins, Philadelphia, PA, USA.

[72] Rao, PS. (2003c) Comparative summary of atrial septal defect occlusion devices, In: *Catheter Based Devices for Treatment of Noncoronary Cardiovascular Disease in Adults and Children,* P.S. Rao, M.J. Kern. (Eds.): 91-101, Lippincott, Williams & Wilkins, Philadelphia, PA, USA.

[73] Rao, PS. (2003d) The buttoned device. In: *Catheter Based Devices for Treatment of Noncoronary Cardiovascular Disease in Adults and Children,* P.S. Rao, M.J. Kern. (Eds.): 17-34, Lippincott, Williams & Wilkins, Philadelphia, PA, USA.

[74] Rao, PS. (2007) Techniques for closure of large atrial septal defects. *Cath Cardiovasc Intervent,* Vol. 70, No. 2, pp. 329-330.

[75] Roman, KS.; Jones, A.; Keeton, BR.; Salmon, AP. (2002) Different techniques for closure of multiple interatrial communications with the Amplatzer septal occluder. *J Interv Cardiol,* Vol. 15, No. 5, pp. 393-397.

[76] Rosas, M.; Attie, F.; Sandoval, J.; et al. (2004) Atrial septal defect in adults ≥40 years old: negative impact of low arterial oxygen saturation. *Int J Cardiol,* Vol. 93, No. 2-3, pp. 145-155.

[77] Salehian, O.; Horlik, E.; Schwermann, M.; et al. (2005) Improvement in cardiac form and function after ttranscatheter closure of secundum atrial septal defects. *J Am Coll Cardiol,* Vol. 45, No. 4, pp. 499-504.

[78] Sievert, H.; Koppeler, P.; Rux, S.; et al. (1999) Percutaneous closure of 176 interatrial defects in adults with different occlusion devices - 6 years experience [abstract]. J Am Coll Cardiol, Vol. 33, No. pp. 519A.

[79] Staniloae, CS.; El-Khally, Z.; Ibrahim, R.; et al. (2003) Percutaneous closure of secondum atrial septal defects in adults – A single center experience with Amplatzer septal occluder. *J Invasive Cardiol,* Vol. 15, No. 7, pp. 393-397.

[80] Szkutnik, M.; Masura, J.; Bialkowski, J.; et al. (2004) Transcatheter Closure of double atrial septal defects with a single Amplatzer device. *Catheter Cardiovasc Intervent,* Vol. 61, No. 2, pp. 237-241.

[81] Tillman, T.; Mulingtapang, R.; Sullebarger, JT. (2008) Approach to percutaneous closure in patients with multiple atrial septal defects. *J Invasive Cardiol,* Vol. 20, No. 5, pp. E167-170.

[82] Varma, C.; Benson, LN.; Silversides, C.; et al. (2004) Outcome and alternative techniques for device closure of large secundum atrial septal defect. *Cath Cardiovasc Intervent,* Vol. 61, No. 1, pp. 131-139.

[83] Walsh, KP.; Tofeig, M.; Kitchiner, DJ.; et al. (1999) Comparison of the Sideris and Amplatzer septal occlusion devices. *Am J Cardiol,* Vol. 83, No. 6, pp. 933-936.

[84] Ward, C. (1994) Secundum atrial septal defect: routine surgical treatment is not of proven benefit. *Br Heart J,* Vol. 71, No. 3, pp. 219–223.

[85] Webb, G. (2001) Do patients over 40 years of age benefit from closure of an atrial septal defect? *Heart,* Vol. 85, No. 3, pp. 249–250.

[86] Zanchetta, M.; Rigatelli, G.; Pedon, L.; et al. (2005) Catheter closure of perforated secundum atrial septal defect under intracardiac echocardiographic guidance using a single Amplatzer device: feasibility of a new method. *J Invasive Cardiol,* Vol. 17, No. 5, pp. 262-265.

9

Atrial Septal Defect Closure in Geriatric Patients

Teiji Akagi
Cardiac Intensive Care Unit, Okayama University Hospital, Okayama, Japan

1. Introduction

The prevalence of adults with congenital heart disease is rising in the general population (1). Similarly, the number of geriatric patients with congenital heart disease, such older than 70 years old, is also rising. Furthermore, mortality rates in congenital heart disease have shifted away from the young and towards adults, with a steady increase in age at death. Actually, the mortality of congenital heart disease in patients whose age 60 years or more is increasing during past few decades reported in Japanese nationwide survey (2). Atrial septal defect (ASD) is the one of the most common congenital heart lesions in adults, and the most influenced heart disease for the death in geriatric population. Prevalence of ASD in children is noted to be 11.4% within the congenital heart defects (3). Majority of these children are asymptomatic and diagnosed by school physical examination, heart murmur detected primary care pediatrician, cardiac echo screening in the newborn period. If defect is smaller than 6 mm, spontaneous closure can be expected. Operation is scheduled based on children's body size, usually before the elementally school with very low incidence of mortality rate (4).

Although the pediatric or young adult ASD population has attracted research interest over the last 2 decades, the geriatric ASD population has yet to be characterized. Extrapolation of studies on younger patients is not appropriate in the geriatric patients. First, geriatric patients with ASD acquire comorbid conditions such as arrhythmia, hypertension, respiratory distress, kidney disease, etc., that always influence on significant role in their heart conditions. Second, geriatric ASD patients may have inherently superior resiliency, milder disease, or balanced physiology in contrast to those not surviving to an advanced age (5). Therefore, geriatric patients with ASD represent a distinct population for which focused studies are needed.

Again, clinical features of atrial septal defect (ASD) in the elderly are significantly different from those in children and young adults. Elderly patients with ASD frequently present with hemodynamic abnormalities such as pulmonary hypertension, atrial arrhythmias, and valvular regurgitation, which cause congestive heart failure. Moreover, various comobidities, such as hypertension, chronic obstructive pulmonary disease, coronary artery disease and left ventricular diastolic dysfunction often complicate the clinical features in this population. Left ventricular diastolic dysfunction, which is also seen as part of normal aging and frequently occurs in elderly individuals with hypertension or increased arterial stiffness [6,7], may cause acute congestive heart failure after ASD closure [8].

After the introduction of Amplatzer Septal Occluder, transcatheter ASD closure has become a well-established treatment for secundum-type ASD, with hemodynamically significant left-to-right shunt in children and young adults. Several studies and our own experience have demonstrated clinical benefits and positive right-heart remodeling, with reduction of the right ventricular end-diastolic diameter.(8-17) However, few studies were published considering geriatric patients, who older than 70 years.(18–21) In this aged population, not only catheter closure of ASD but also surgical closure has been reported very limited experiences, little data are published on functional results. In this chapter, I would like to report our current experience of catheter closure of ASD in geriatric patients (70 years or more), and its long-term outcome.

2. Patient's background

From 2005 to 2010, transcatheter closure of ASD was attempted in 420 patients in our hospital. Of those patients, 30 patients who were older than 70 years were retrospectively assessed. Patient characteristics, clinical, hemodynamic and echocardiographic data, and ASD morphology are shown in Table 1. There were 10 males and 20 females with a mean

Total patients	*30*
Gender, F/M	*20/10*
Age, (range), yrs	*75.8 ± 3.8 (70-85)*
BSA, m^2	*1.5 ± 0.2*
Hypertension	*12 (40%)*
Stroke	*4 (13%)*
CAD	*2 (7%)*
COPD	*5 (17%)*
Atrial fibrillation	*16 (53%)*
Paroxysmal	*3 (10%)*
Permanent	*13 (43%)*
RBBB	*22 (74%)*
*Systolic PAP *, mmHg*	*35.6 ± 11.8*
PAH	*16 (53%)*
E', cm/s	*7.1 ± 1.9*
E/E`	*11.0 ± 3.9*
Diuretic use	*17 (57%)*
Hospitarization for HF	*9 (30%)*
NYHA functional class, I / II / III	*5 /17 / 8*
*Qp/Qs**	*2.4 ± 0.7*
ASD size, mm	*20.3 ± 6.4*
Rim type	
Sufficient rim, n (%)	*8 (27%)*
Aortic rim deficient, n (%)	*19 (63%)*
Aortic and anterosuperior rim deficient, n (%)	*1 (3%)*
IVC rim deficient, n (%)	*2 (7%)*

BSA, body surface area; CAD, coronary artery disease; COPD, chronic obstructive pulmonary disease
RBBB, right bundle branch block; PAP, pulmonary artery pressure; PAH, pulmonary artery hypertension
E, early diastolic mitral valve flow velocity; E', early diastolic mitral annular velocity; HF, heart failure
NYHA, New York Heart Association; Qp, pulmonary flow; Qs, systemic flow; IVC, inferior vena cava

Table 1. Patients Characteristics

age of 75.8 ± 3.8 years and age range of 70 to 85 years. Eighteen of the 30 patients had been diagnosed with ASD within 2 years before transcatheter closure was attempted but the others well before that. Most of the patients had at least one major comorbidity, including systemic hypertension, stroke, coronary artery disease, and atrial fibrillation. Mean systolic pulmonary artery pressure at the time of diagnostic catheterization was 35.6 ± 11.8 mmHg. Mean early diastolic mitral annular velocity (e') and the ratio of early diastolic mitral valve flow velocity (E) to e' (E/e') suggested that our cohort generally had impaired myocardial relaxation.(22,23) Twelve patients had been diagnosed with ASD well before transcatheter closure was attempted but they had refused or hesitated to receive ASD closure. We think that this was partially because they had no recognizable symptom, but mainly because surgical closure was the only treatment at the time when they had been first diagnosed with ASD. More than half of the patients were being treated with a diuretic for congestive heart failure, and 30% of the patients had a history of hospitalization due to heart failure. Seventeen patients were classified as NYHA functional class II and 8 patients were classified as class III. Only 5 patients had no symptoms despite significant shunt flow and were classified as NYHA functional class I. One patient had two defects. Mean defect diameter was 20.3 ± 6.4 mm, and a circumferentially sufficient rim (> 5 mm rim around the defect) was observed in only 8 patients. Mean pulmonary-systemic flow ratio (Qp/Qs) calculated by using the Fick principle was 2.4 ± 0.7.

3. Hemodynamic features during ASD closure in geriatric patients

Previous studies have suggested that development of acute congestive heart failure is due to abrupt elevation in left ventricular preload following transcatheter ASD closure, especially in elderly patients with impaired left ventricular systolic or diastolic function (6,24,25) In our experience, despite the fact that our patients had impaired left ventricular diastolic function estimated by decreased e' and increased E/e' (23,26) as well as various comorbidities such as systemic hypertension, pulmonary artery hypertension and atrial fibrillation, acute congestive heart failure after the ASD closure did not develop in any of the patients except in one patient in whom the procedure was abandoned due to PCWP elevation during test balloon occlusion. Schubert et al. reported that peri-procedural anticongestive medication was effective in preventing congestive heart failure after ASD closure in elderly patients (27). In our experience, 57% of the 30 patients previously used oral diuretics, and this high rate of diuretic usage might have contributed to prevention of acute congestive heart failure after closure.

4. Transcatheter ASD closure

Transcatheter ASD closure was conducted under general anesthesia with the guidance of fluoroscopy and TEE. Amplatzer® Septal Occluder (St. Jude Medical, St. Paul, MN) was used for all closures, and the procedure was performed as previously described (28). For patients who had a history of heart failure and were considered to be hemodynamically high-risk, we placed a Swan-Ganz catheter into pulmonary artery from the internal jugular vein or femoral vein and monitored pulmonary artery wedge pressure (PCWP) during subsequent procedure. If mean PCWP increased > 5 mmHg from the baseline value during balloon occlusion of the defect (test balloon occlusion), we judged the procedure should not be indicated. (Fig. 1) Medications such as diuretics, warfarin, and antihypertension and antiarrhythmia drugs were continued at the same doses after the procedure.

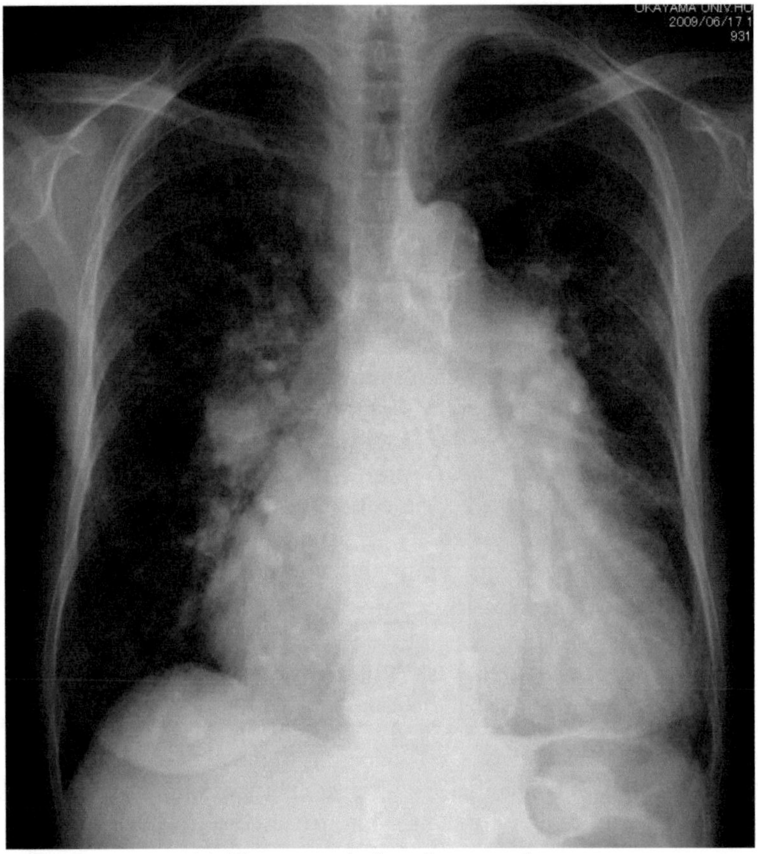

(a) Chest x ray before the procedure

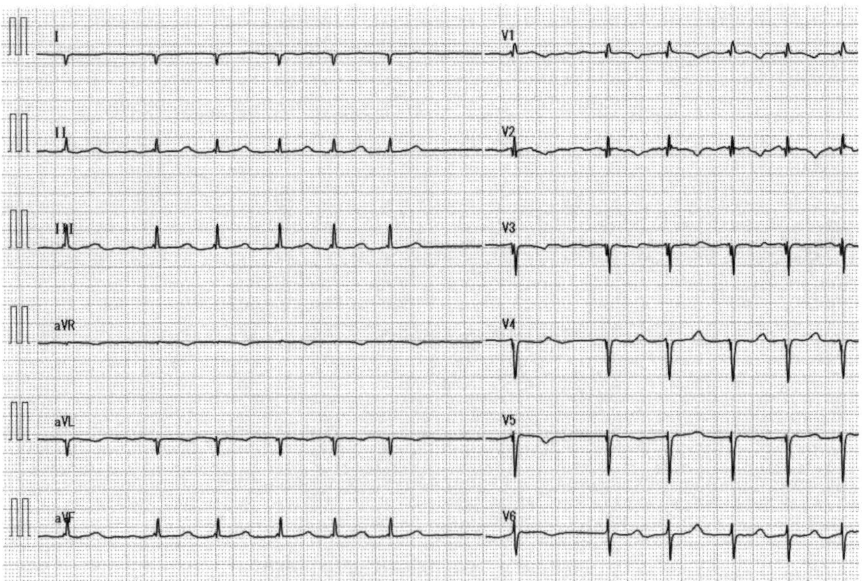

(b) ECG finings before the procedure

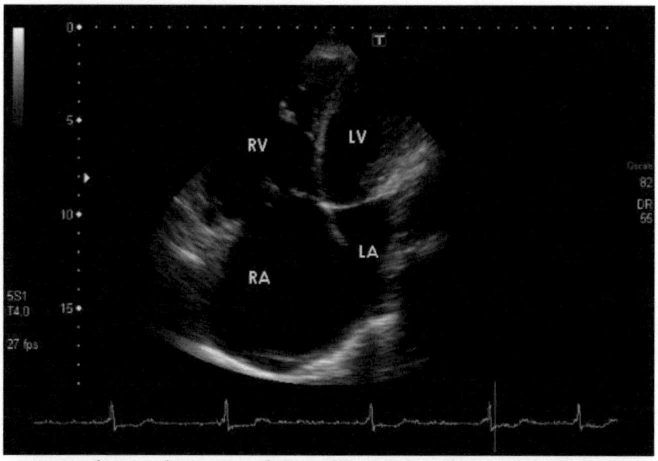

(c) apical 4 chamber view of transthoracic echocardiography: RA and RV are significantly enlarged

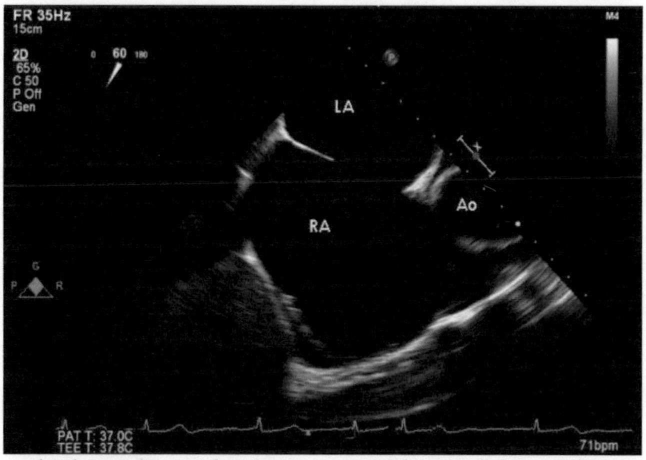

(d) transesophageal echocardiography demonstrated 30mm defect with aortic rim deficiency

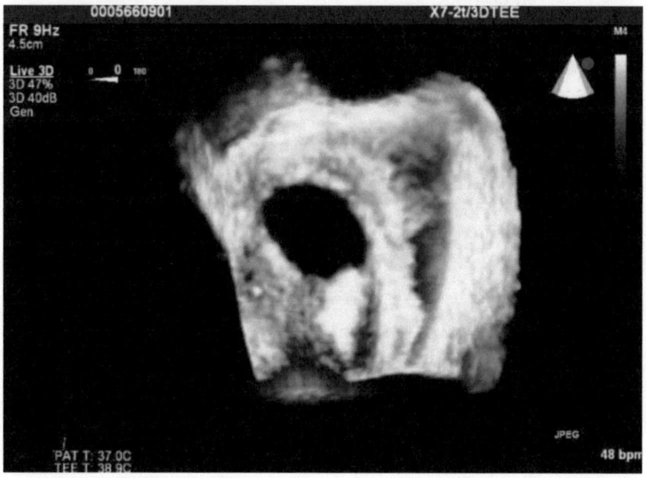

(e) 3d transesophageal echocardiography demonstrated the elliptical shape of ASD

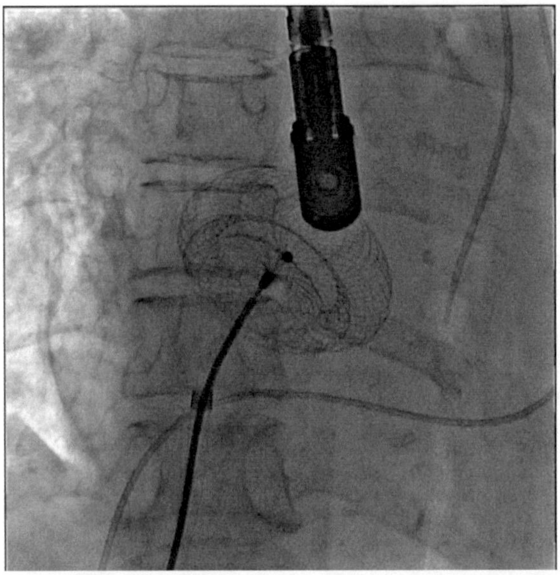

(f) Catheter closure of ASD using 34mm device, PCW pressure monitored continuously

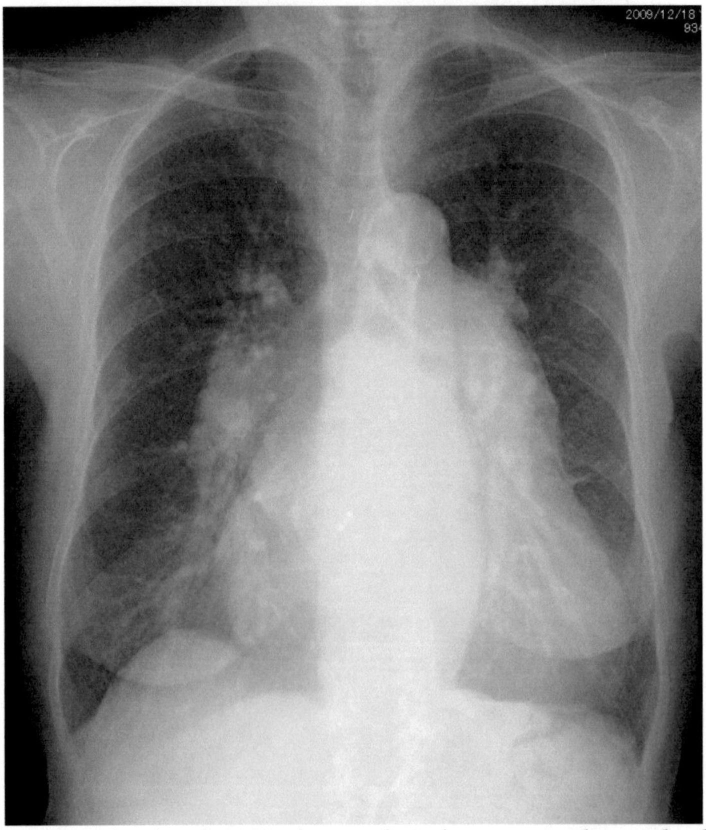

(g) Chest x-ray 6 months after the ASD closure, clinical symptoms also resolved completely

Fig. 1. 82 years old female, ASD with permanent atrial fibrillation.

Prior to ASD closure, test balloon occlusion were performed in 7 of 30 cases. As a result, the procedure was abandoned in one case due to a significant elevation of PCWP during test occlusion of the ASD. This patient was an 84-year-old thin woman who had permanent atrial fibrillation, hypertension, chronic kidney disease, chronic anemia and severe TR. She had been repeatedly hospitalized with congestive heart failure in past years. Her ASD diameter was 24 mm and Qp/Qs was 2.6. During test balloon occlusion, her PCWP immediately increased from 8 mmHg to 22 mmHg and remained at 16 mmHg after 20 minutes, thus procedure was abandoned. In the other 2 cases, the device was difficult to deploy because of large size defect. One of those cases proceeded to surgical closure, and the other case was successfully closed in the second attempt of catheter intervention on a later day. Finally, 28 (93%) of the 30 patients were treated successfully by catheter closure. A single device was placed in 27 patients. In the remaining patient with multiple defects, 2 devices were deployed at the time of the same procedure. Mean device diameter was 23.3 ± 6.0 mm. Mean follow-up period was 19.1 ± 11.3 months.

5. Procedural outcomes

Table 2 shows the procedural and mid-term results. Device closure was successfully performed in 28 (93%) of the 30 patients without acute complications. In the other 2 patients, the procedures were abandoned because of technical issues. While only 8 (27%) of the 30 patients had sufficient rim type ASD, 19 (63%) had aortic rim deficient type. However, there was not much difference in our device selection between sufficient rim and aortic rim deficient type. Therefore, we think that the small percentage of patients with sufficient rim did not have a great impact on device size selection in the present study. Although the majority of our patients were complicated with various comorbidities, such as pulmonary artery hypertension, systemic hypertension and atrial fibrillation, high procedural success rate can be expected even in this aged group. Also, significant improvement of NYHA functional class was observed after closure even though about 30% of the patients in this

Procedural results (n=30)	
Success deployment, n (%)	*28 (93%)*
Device size, mm	*23.3 ± 6.0*
Acute complication, n (%)	*0 (0%)*
Mid-term results (n=28)	
Meam follow-up period, m	*19.1 ± 11.3*
Residual shunt, n (%)	*2 (8%)*
Major events	
Death, n (%)	*2 (8%)*
sudden death, n	*1 (4%)**
prostate cancer, n	*1 (4%)*
Pacemaker implantation, n (%)	*1 (4%)*
TIA, n (%)	*1 (4%)**
Persistent AF, n (%)	*1 (4%)*
	** the same case*

TIA, transient ischemic attack; AF, atrial fibrillation

Table 2. Procedural and Mid-term Results

study had a history of hospitalization for congestive heart failure. No patient required additional hospitalization for congestive heart failure during the follow-up period. The first procedure was successful in 27 of 30 cases in which transcatheter ASD closure was attempted. On the other hand, the procedure was abandoned in 3 cases.

Two patients died during the follow-up period. One died of prostatic cancer 20 months after ASD closure. The other patient died 2 months after the procedure. This patient was a 70-year-old woman who had permanent atrial fibrillation, severe chronic obstructive pulmonary disease, mild left ventricular dysfunction, history of pacemaker implantation for sick sinus syndrome, and mitral valve replacement and was in NYHA functional class III. Her ASD was 22 mm with a sufficient atrial rim, and a 26 mm device was used for closure. She died from unknown cause at home; however, a history of transient cerebral ischemic attack was reported one week before her death. Autopsy was not performed. During the follow-up period, 3 complications occurred. One patient who was complicated with several cardiac comorbidities died 2 months after the procedure. An autopsy was not performed and it was therefore not known whether the cause of sudden death was ASD device-associated.

6. Atrial arrhythmias

Two patients were complicated with new arrhythmia. One patient who had permanent atrial fibrillation underwent pacemaker implantation for slow ventricular response 6 months after ASD closure. The other patient with paroxysmal atrial fibrillation before ASD closure developed persistent atrial fibrillation during the follow-up period. The remaining 24 patients had no late complication during the follow-up period. No patient had hemodynamically significant residual shunt.

Table 3 shows time course changes in clinical and echocardiographic parameters. Follow-up data (at more than 6 months after the procedure) were available in all of the 28 patients with exception of one patient who died 2 months after the procedure. NYHA functional class was significantly improved in 20 (74%) of the 27 patients at the latest follow-up (Fig. 2). One patient who remained in NYHA class III was complicated with severe chronic obstructive pulmonary disease. There was also a significant improvement in plasma BNP level (175.9 ± 64.7 vs. 99.2 ± 83.2 pg/ml, P=0.013). Resting heart rate also decreased significantly (74.4 ± 14.5 vs. 66.7 ± 8.7 beats/min, P=0.005), although no cardiac chronotropic drug was administered to any of the patients. Pacemaker implantation was required in one patient 6 months after the procedure, even though bradycardia was not observed before or just after ASD closure. In one patient, paroxysmal atrial fibrillation progressed into persistent atrial fibrillation 2 years after ASD closure. In previous studies, the incidence of atrial fibrillation in patients after transcatheter ASD closure was estimated to be 5% to 18% (29-31), however, especially in elderly patients, atrial fibrillation is one of the expected findings for their natural course after ASD closure.

7. Cardiac remodeling

RVEDD and estimated systolic pulmonary artery pressure decreased significantly (40.8 ± 6.0 vs. 31.6 ± 4.5 mm, P<0.001, 38.5 ± 12.7 vs. 27.2 ± 7.3 mmHg, P<0.001, respectively). At the

	Pre-procedure (n=27)	Follow-up (n=27)	p Value
NYHA functional class, n (%)			< 0.001
I	3 (11%)	21 (78%)	
II	17 (63%)	5 (18%)	
III	7 (26%)	1 (4%)	
Plasma BNP level, pg/mL	175.9 ± 249.7	99.2 ± 83.2	0.013
HR at rest, bpm	74.4 ± 14.5	66.7 ± 8.7	0.005
Estimate systolic PAP, mmHg	38.5 ± 12.7	27.2 ± 7.3	< 0.001
RVEDD, mm	40.8 ± 6.0	31.6 ± 4.5	< 0.001
LVEDD mm	39.7 ± 4.8	45.3 ± 4.6	< 0.001
RVEDD/LVEDD ratio	1.05 ± 0.24	0.70 ± 0.12	< 0.001
LAD, mm	46.1 ± 9.9	44.3 ± 9.3	0.128
LVEF, %	70.5 ± 6.1	70.5 ± 5.7	0.611
TR, n (%)			0.002
≤ mild	10 (37%)	20 (74%)	
moderate	13 (48%)	7 (26%)	
severe	4 (15%)	0 (0%)	
MR, n (%)			0.004
none or trivial	18 (67%)	8 (30%)	
mild	6 (22%)	16 (59%)	
> moderate	3 (11%)	3 (11%)	

BNP, brain natriuretic peptide; PAP, pulmonary artery pressure; RVEDD, right ventricular end-diastolic dimension; LAD, left ventricular dimension; LVEF, left ventricular ejection fraction; TR, tricuspid regurgitation; MR, mitral regurgitation

Table 3. Changes of Clinical Echocardiographic Parameters

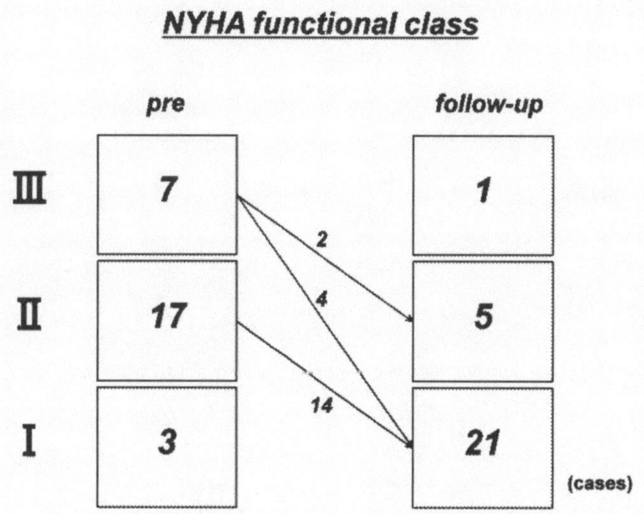

Fig. 2. NYHA functional class before the procedure and at follow-up.

same time, LVEDD increased significantly (39.7 ± 4.8 vs. 45.3 ± 4.6 mm, P<0.001). Therefore, the RVEDD/LVEDD ratio significantly decreased (1.05 ± 0.24 vs. 0.70 ± 0.12 mm, reduction of 67%, P<0.001), indicating ventricular reverse remodeling. Left atrial dimension, above the normal level at baseline, did not change significantly during the follow-up period. Left ventricular ejection fraction also did not change. During the follow-up period, NYHA functional class significantly improved in 20 (74%) of the 27 patients. Our data also demonstrated significant decreases of heart rate, pulmonary artery pressure and plasma BNP level, and these changes contributed to the improvement of NYHA functional class. Decrement of heart rate is presumably evidence of increment of left ventricular stroke volume following increased left ventricular preload after abolishment of left-to-right shunt. Significant decrease in RVEDD/LVEDD ratio was observed even in our geriatric patients, although RVEDD did not reach the normal level. Interestingly, percentage change in RVEDD/LVEDD ratio in our cohort was equivalent to results of other studies in younger populations (25,32). Furthermore, it was revealed that RVEDD/LVEDD ratio was independently correlated with NYHA functional class in the follow-up period.

8. AV valve regurgitation

Improvement of TR was observed in 11 of 17 patients (65%) with moderate or severe degree of regurgitation during the follow-up period (Fig. 3). On the other hand, MR was increased in 10 (37%) of the 27 patients and was unchanged in the others (63%) during the follow-up period (Fig. 4). In our cohort, there was no patient with mitral valve prolapse as a cause for MR. In this study, the degree of TR was decreased in 11 patients (41%) and exacerbation of

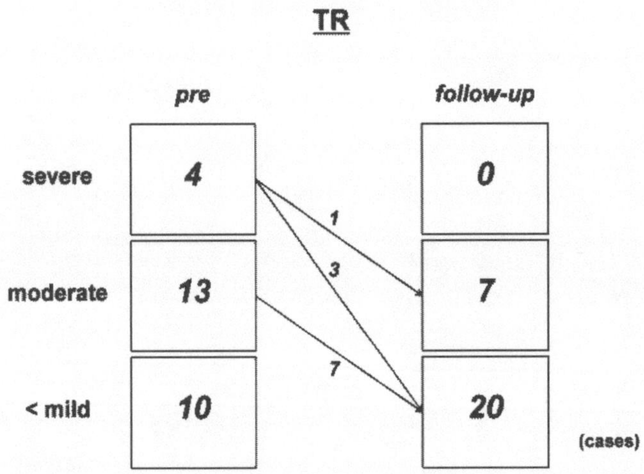

Fig. 3. Degrees of TR before the procedure and at follow-up.

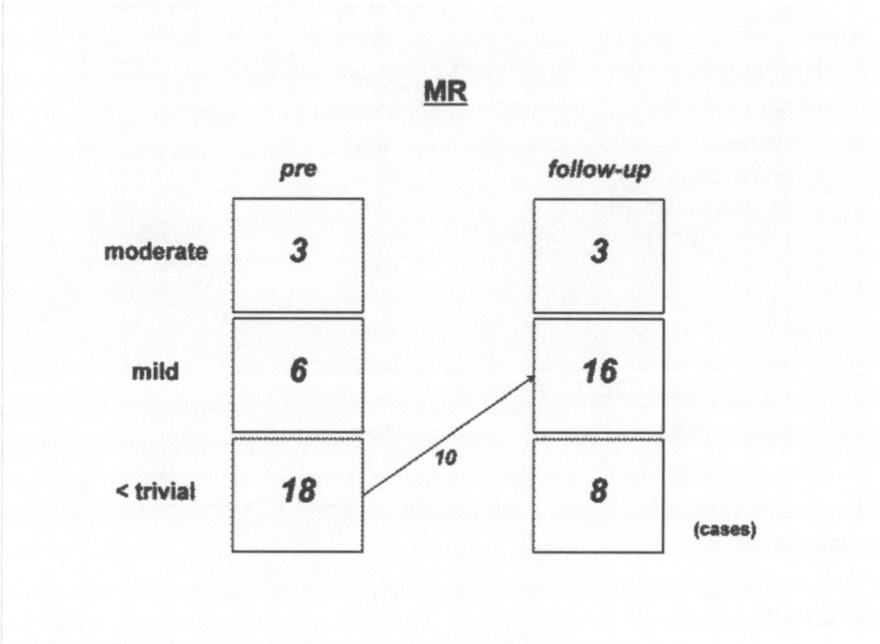

Fig. 4. Degrees of MR before the procedure and at follow-up.

TR was not observed during the follow-up period. Interestingly, in the case of moderate or severe TR before ASD closure, the degree of TR was improved in 11 (65%) of the 17 patients. TR can be improved functionally following decrement of right ventricular preload after ASD closure. Improvement of TR also can be expected following improvement of right ventricular geometric abnormality (33,34). Our results suggest that TR can be improved even in geriatric patients and that the severity of TR does not become a factor to exclude them as candidates for transcatheter ASD closure. On the other hand, the degree of MR was slightly increased in 10 patients (37%) and unchanged in the others (63%) during the follow-up period. Wilson et al. reported that the degree of MR was unchanged in 83% and increased in 10% of their 194 patients, including 78 patients aged younger than 15 years, after transcatheter ASD closure (35). In elderly ASD patients, the severity of MR might be masked by the presence of ASD effectively reducing left ventricular preload. Additionally, degenerated change of the mitral valve leaflet also influenced the increase in MR. Although the degree of MR and the increase in MR were not associated with NYHA functional class in the follow-up period in our study, further long-term follow-up is mandatory.

Associations between NYHA functional class and echocardiographic parameters in the follow-up period

Table 4 shows associations of clinical and echocardiographic parameters with NYHA functional class. In the follow-up period, RVEDD/LVEDD ratio was identified as a factor associated with NYHA functional class. On the other hand, E/e', e', degree of TR or MR and increase in MR were not associated with NYHA functional class.

Variable	r	Univariate p Value	Multivariate p Value
Age		0.349	
Qp/Qs		0.807	
HR at rest		0.260	
plasma BNP level		0.146	
Estimate systolic PAP		0.382	
RVEDD/LVEDD ratio	0.491	0.009	0.009
LVEF, %		0.971	
E/e'		0.688	
e'		0.962	
Degree of TR		0.282	
Degree of MR		0.682	
increase in MR		0.764	

Table 4. Association betwwen Clinical and Echocardiographic Parameters and NYHA class at Follow-up Period

9. Conclusions

Although our experience is still small, even in elderly patients older than 70 years, transcatheter closure of ASD can be performed safely and contributes to significant improvement of NYHA functional class and positive cardiac remodeling. Further investigation is required especially for the outcome of MR

10. References

[1] Afilalo J, Therrien J, Pilote L, at al. Geriatric congenital heart disease: burden of disease and predictors of mortality. J. Am. Coll. Cardiol. 2011;58;1509-1515

[2] Terai M, Niwa K, Nakazawa M, Tatsuno K, Segami K, Hamada H, Kohno Y, Oki I, Nakamura Y. Mortality from congenital cardiovascular malformations in Japan, 1968 through 1997. Circ J. 2002;66:484-8.

[3] Sama´nek M, Slavis Z, Zborilova´ B, Hrobonova´ V, Voriskova´ M, Skovra´nek J. Prevalence, treatment and outcome of heart disease in live-born children: a prospective analysis of 91,823 live-born children. Pediatr Cardiol. 1989;10:205–211.

[4] Radzik D, Davignon A, van Doesburg N, Fournier A, Marchand T, Ducharme G. Predictive factors for spontaneous closure of atrial septal defects diagnosed in the first 3 months of life. J Am Coll Cardiol. 1993;22:851-3.

[5] Report of the British Cardiac Society Working Party. Grown-up congenital heart (GUCH) disease: current needs and provision of service for adolescents and adults with congenital heart disease in the UK. Heart 2002;88 Suppl 1:i1–14.

[6] Abhayaratna WP, Marwick TH, Smith WT, Becker NG. Characteristics of left ventricular diastolic dysfunction in the community: an echocardiographic survey. Heart 2006;92:1259-1264.

[7] Vasan RS, Benjamin EJ, Levy D. Prevalence, clinical features and prognosis of diastolic heart failure: an epidemiologic perspective. J Am Coll Cardiol 1995;26:1565-1574.

[8] Ewert P, Berger F, Nagdyman N, Kretschmar O, Dittrich S, Abdul-Khaliq H, Lange P. Masked left ventricular restriction in elderly patients with atrial septal defects: a contraindication for closure? Catheter Cardiovasc Interv 2001;52:177-180.
[9] Chan KC, Godman MJ, Walsh K, Wilson N, Redington A, Gibbs JL. Transcatheter closure of atrial septal defect and interatrial communications with a new self expanding nitinol double disc device (Amplatzer septal occluder): multicentre UK experience. Heart 1999;82:300-306.
[10] Santoro G, Pascotto M, Caputo S, Cerrato F, Cappelli Bigazzi M, Palladino MT, Iacono C, Carrozza M, Russo MG, Calabro R. Similar cardiac remodelling after transcatheter atrial septal defect closure in children and young adults. Heart 2006;92:958-962.
[11] Du ZD, Koenig P, Cao QL, Waight D, Heitschmidt M, Hijazi ZM. Comparison of transcatheter closure of secundum atrial septal defect using the Amplatzer septal occluder associated with deficient versus sufficient rims. Am J Cardiol 2002;90:865-869.
[12] Wu ET, Akagi T, Taniguchi M, Maruo T, Sakuragi S, Otsuki S, Okamoto Y, Sano S. Differences in right and left ventricular remodeling after transcatheter closure of atrial septal defect among adults. Catheter Cardiovasc Interv 2007;69:866-871.
[13] Schoen SP, Kittner T, Bohl S, Braun MU, Simonis G, Schmeisser A, Strasser RH. Transcatheter closure of atrial septal defects improves right ventricular volume, mass, function, pulmonary pressure, and functional class: a magnetic resonance imaging study. Heart 2006;92:821-826.
[14] Spies C, Khandelwal A, Timmermanns I, Schrader R. Incidence of atrial fibrillation following transcatheter closure of atrial septal defects in adults. Am J Cardiol 2008;102:902-906.
[15] Salehian O, Horlick E, Schwerzmann M, Haberer K, McLaughlin P, Siu SC, Webb G, Therrien J. Improvements in cardiac form and function after transcatheter closure of secundum atrial septal defects. J Am Coll Cardiol 2005;45:499-504.
[16] Masura J, Gavora P, Podnar T. Long-term outcome of transcatheter secundum-type atrial septal defect closure using Amplatzer septal occluders. J Am Coll Cardiol 2005;45:505-507.
[17] Jategaonkar S, Scholtz W, Schmidt H, Horstkotte D. Percutaneous closure of atrial septal defects: echocardiographic and functional results in patients older than 60 years. Circ Cardiovasc Interv 2009;2:85-89.
[18] Elshershari H, Cao QL, Hijazi ZM. Transcatheter device closure of atrial septal defects in patients older than 60 years of age: immediate and follow-up results. J Invasive Cardiol 2008;20:173-176.
[19] Khan AA, Tan JL, Li W, Dimopoulos K, Spence MS, Chow P, Mullen MJ. The impact of transcatheter atrial septal defect closure in the older population: a prospective study. JACC Cardiovasc Interv 2010;3:276-281.
[20] Taniguchi M, Akagi T, Ohtsuki S, Okamoto Y, Tanabe Y, Watanabe N, Nakagawa K, Toh N, Kusano K, Sano S. Transcatheter closure of atrial septal defect in elderly patients with permanent atrial fibrillation. Catheter Cardiovasc Interv 2009;73:682-686.
[21] Nakagawa K, Akagi T, Taniguchi M, et. Al. Transcatheter Closure of Atrial Septal Defect in a Geriatric Population. Catheter Cardiovasc Interv 2012 (in press)
[22] Miyatake K, Izumi S, Okamoto M, Kinoshita N, Asonuma H, Nakagawa H, Yamamoto K, Takamiya M, Sakakibara H, Nimura Y. Semiquantitative grading of severity of

mitral regurgitation by real-time two-dimensional Doppler flow imaging technique. J Am Coll Cardiol 1986;7:82-88.
[23] Sohn DW, Chai IH, Lee DJ, Kim HC, Kim HS, Oh BH, Lee MM, Park YB, Choi YS, Seo JD, Lee YW. Assessment of mitral annulus velocity by Doppler tissue imaging in the evaluation of left ventricular diastolic function. J Am Coll Cardiol 1997;30:474-480.
[24] Tomai F, Ando G, De Paulis R, Chiariello L. Real-time evaluation of the hemodynamic effects of atrial septal defect closure in adults with left ventricular dysfunction. Catheter Cardiovasc Interv 2005;64:124-126.
[25] Holzer R, Cao QL, Hijazi ZM. Closure of a moderately large atrial septal defect with a self-fabricated fenestrated Amplatzer septal occluder in an 85-year-old patient with reduced diastolic elasticity of the left ventricle. Catheter Cardiovasc Interv 2005;64:513-8; discussion 519-521.
[26] Ommen SR, Nishimura RA, Appleton CP, Miller FA, Oh JK, Redfield MM, Tajik AJ. Clinical utility of Doppler echocardiography and tissue Doppler imaging in the estimation of left ventricular filling pressures: A comparative simultaneous Doppler-catheterization study. Circulation 2000;102:1788-1794.
[27] Schubert S, Peters B, Abdul-Khaliq H, Nagdyman N, Lange PE, Ewert P. Left ventricular conditioning in the elderly patient to prevent congestive heart failure after transcatheter closure of atrial septal defect. Catheter Cardiovasc Interv 2005;64:333-337.
[28] Thanopoulos BD, Laskari CV, Tsaousis GS, Zarayelyan A, Vekiou A, Papadopoulos GS. Closure of atrial septal defects with the Amplatzer occlusion device: preliminary results. J Am Coll Cardiol 1998;31:1110-1116.
[29] Berger F, Vogel M, Alexi-Meskishvili V, Lange PE. Comparison of results and complications of surgical and Amplatzer device closure of atrial septal defects. J Thorac Cardiovasc Surg 1999;118:674-8; discussion 678-680.
[30] Silversides CK, Siu SC, McLaughlin PR, Haberer KL, Webb GD, Benson L, Harris L. Symptomatic atrial arrhythmias and transcatheter closure of atrial septal defects in adult patients. Heart 2004;90:1194-1198.
[31] Oliver JM, Gallego P, Gonzalez A, Benito F, Mesa JM, Sobrino JA. Predisposing conditions for atrial fibrillation in atrial septal defect with and without operative closure. Am J Cardiol 2002;89:39-43.
[32] Du ZD, Hijazi ZM, Kleinman CS, Silverman NH, Larntz K. Comparison between transcatheter and surgical closure of secundum atrial septal defect in children and adults: results of a multicenter nonrandomized trial. J Am Coll Cardiol 2002;39:1836-1844.
[33] Berger M, Haimowitz A, Van Tosh A, Berdoff RL, Goldberg E. Quantitative assessment of pulmonary hypertension in patients with tricuspid regurgitation using continuous wave Doppler ultrasound. J Am Coll Cardiol 1985;6:359-365.
[34] Toyono M, Krasuski RA, Pettersson GB, Matsumura Y, Yamano T, Shiota T. Persistent tricuspid regurgitation and its predictor in adults after percutaneous and isolated surgical closure of secundum atrial septal defect. Am J Cardiol 2009;104:856-861.
[35] Wilson NJ, Smith J, Prommete B, O'Donnell C, Gentles TL, Ruygrok PN. Transcatheter closure of secundum atrial septal defects with the Amplatzer septal occluder in adults and children-follow-up closure rates, degree of mitral regurgitation and evolution of arrhythmias. Heart Lung Circ 2008;17:318-324.

Section 6

Patent Foramen Ovale

10

Atrial Septal Defect/Patent Foramen Ovale and Migraine Headache

Mohammed Tawfiq Numan
University of Texas, Houston, Texas
USA

1. Introduction

Migraine headaches affect approximately 13% of US population, affecting women in a 3:1 ratio and with a 60-80% familial inheritance. Migraine is a relevant social health problem; in fact it significantly restricts the social life of those who are affected. Recently, migraine headache has been suspected to be a potential risk factor for stroke, particularly in women, smokers and for those making use of oral contraception.

Onset of migraine is usually between the ages of 20-64, with over 80% having their first episode before age 30 and tends to decrease in middle age. Migraine with aura (MA) is a variant characterized by transient neurological visual, verbal, sensory or motor symptoms that last from five to sixty minutes. MA is also known as "classic migraine" though only 25% of migraneurs experience an aura.

Increased frequency of patent foramen Ovale (PFO) in migraneurs was first reported in 1998 in a case-control study.

An increased prevalence between patent foramen Ovale (PFOs) and migraine exists but there is conflicting data of a causal relationship between these two conditions. It remains controversial whether cardiac screening and intervention provides a treatment benefit in migraneurs and is an area currently investigated for demonstrating clinical benefit of PFO closure. This topic is an intersection between the practice of primary care physicians, neurologists, and cardiologists on the best practice and management of patients with difficult to control migraines given the billions spent on physician visits and pharmacotherapy.

Several mechanisms linking PFO to migraine have been hypothesized, including humoral causes (serotonin-platelet activation, aggregation, and embolism causing cortical spreading depression) and genetic causes (autosomal dominant inheritance with incomplete penetrance). The presence of a right to left shunt (RLS) may be the most potent trigger of migraine attacks with or without aura, and researchers have speculated that a large RLS may contribute to the high risk of ischemic stroke in migraneurs with PFO.

Diagnostic Modalities to evaluate the presence or absence of PFO in the migraine patients are another controversial subject. Mostly agree that the Trans -thoracic echocardiography is less sensitive test particularly in adolescents and adults. Trans- Esophageal and Intra-Cardiac Echocardiography carry more reliability in detecting left to right shunt. Recently Trans-Cranial Doppler has been postulated as more accurate test to detect the right to left shunting in those patients.

PFO closure (particularly device closure) carries the most controversial issue in this subject. With only –so far- one randomized large clinical trial and several prospective cohorts and case control studies, there is conflicting data about the benefit of PFO closure in relieving or treating the Migraine headache.

This chapter will talk first about the anatomy and physiology of Patent Foramen Ovale in normal population, anatomical variants of the PFO, the current diagnostic methods used by different institutions then seeks to summarize the current literature on the association of PFO and migraine headache and studies that have investigated PFO closure in this population.

1.1 Definitions

The topic of Migraine headache in association with Patent Foramen Ovale (PFO) has been one of the controversial topics in the literature. Since 1998 when the first scientific observation that patients with migraine headaches have higher prevelance of PFO(1), the dogma between causation, association and prevention has continued.

In order to make reading through this chapter easier, some definitions will be instated:

2. Patent foramen ovale in normal population

Several studies reported high prevalence of PFO in normal subjects. The highest prevalence reported was in autopsy studies. With a probe inserted in the region of the foremen ovale, if the probe can be passed through it then he/she will be labeled to have PFO. Such studies reported incidence of 25% (2). While looking for the incidence of PFO in Normal population by Trans Esophageal Echocardiogram reported to be less than autopsy studies about 15% (3-4).

The foramen ovale is composed of the septum primum and the septum secundum joined in parallel, forming a tunnel-like structure allowing the oxygenated blood from the placenta to pass towards the systemic circulation. Postnatally, it closes with a valve-like mechanism. Patent foramen ovale results from lack of post neonatal closure. Under certain hemodynamic conditions, when there is a transient pressure gradient from the right to left atria, a PFO can open and enable blood or any blood borne substances to pass from the venous to the arterial circulation. This process is the mechanism of paradoxical embolism, which has been frequently reported in the literature (5-8). There are multiple anatomical variants of PFO morphology (figure 1). Occasionally the PFO has an association with atrial septal aneurysm (figure 2). These variants and atrial aneurysm has been believed to play a major role of the amount and the direction of shunt across the PFO.

3. Migraine headache

Migraine is a common, disabling, largely inherited neurological disorder with a prevalence of 8% to 13% in the population of the Western hemisphere (9, 10), with a 3:1 female preponderance.

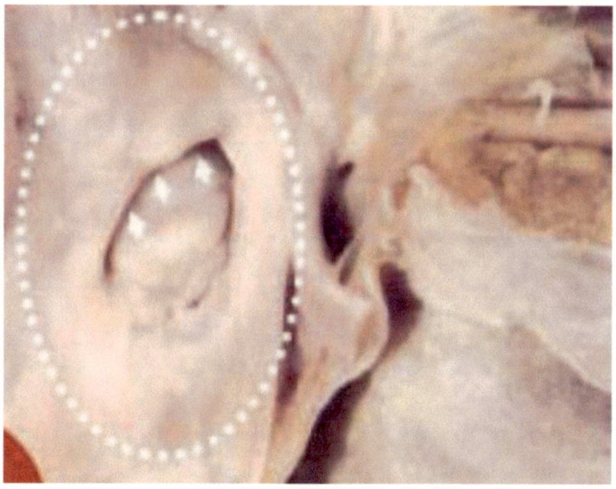

(a)

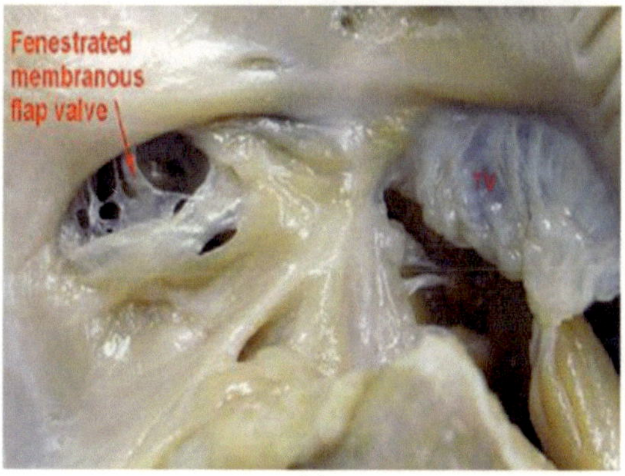

(b)

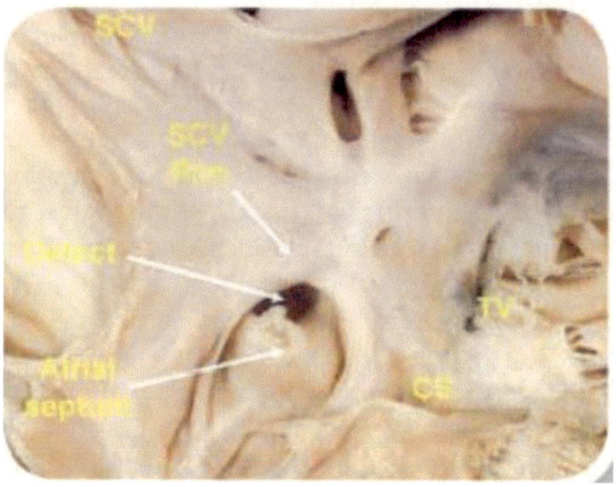

(c)

Fig. 1. Several Morphologies of Patent Foramen Ovale. a: the common type of PFO with a tunnel (white arrows) that can stretch with Valsava. b: Multi fenestration defects in the PFO region. c: a deficient part of the secundum septum covering the PFO from the left side of the atrial septum.

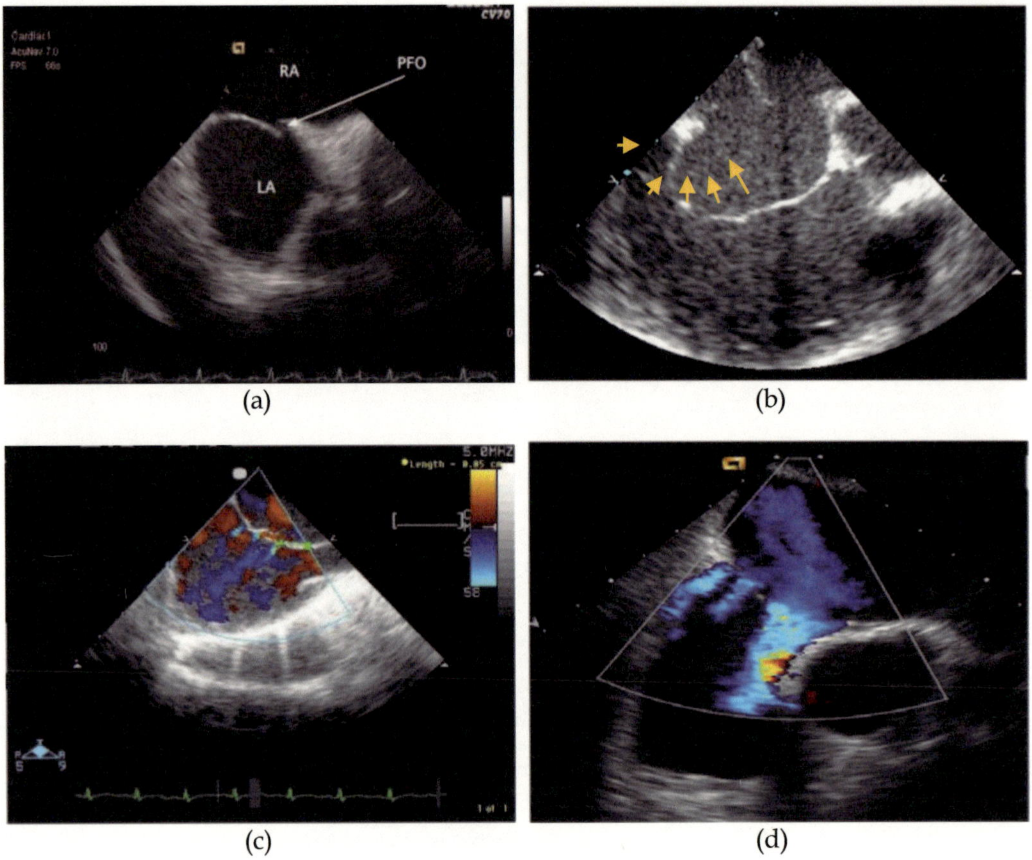

Fig. 2. Echocardiographic appearance of different PFO morphologies, a: Intra Cardiac Echo (ICE) of a tunnel shape PFO. b: Large atrial aneurysm (orange arrow heads) by trans thoracic echo(TTE). c: small multi fenestration by TTE color Doppler. d: larger fenestrations by TEE color Doppler.

Migraine is a common, chronic, disabling neurovascular disorder characterized by attacks of severe headache, autonomic nervous system dysfunction, and, in some patients, an aura and neurological symptoms (11). The suffering associated with migraine headaches accounts for a significant loss in productivity and a substantial increase in healthcare-related costs. About 60% of the patients with Migraine reported that they can't go to work while having the headache. In approximately one third of sufferers, an aura—consisting of reversible neurological symptoms such as visual illusions, unilateral paresthesias, and expressive/receptive language dysfunction—will precede or occur during some attacks. A typical migraneurs has one to two attacks per month, with a median duration of 24 hours. In addition, approximately 2% of the population experiences a more disabling form of migraine, known as chronic migraine, which is characterized by headache on more than 15 days/month.

The diagnosis of migraine is purely clinical, and its physiopathology is complex and not fully understood, with both genetic and environmental factors appearing to play an important role. Genetic effects, including autosomal dominant inheritance with incomplete penetrance (12, 15) and coinheritance, (13) have also been reported.

The prevailing hypothesis regarding the pathogenesis of migraine is an inherited excitability of certain brain networks that, when triggered by particular endogenous or exogenous factors, leads to a cascade of events that result in head pain, in addition to a multitude of other symptoms, including a heightened sensitivity to movement and ambient light, noise, and odor; nausea; emesis; cognitive impairment; vertigo; depression; and lethargy (14). Commonly used preventive medications such as Propranolol, Amitryptiline or anticonvulsants reduce headache frequency in the range of 30-50%, as compared to placebo (16-17).

Migraine occurs in about 15% of the pediatric population, with approximately

One-third of cases associated with an aura (18).

3.1 The association of migraine headache and patent foramen ovale

The initial observation of this association came from the studies of vascular embolic strokes and PFO. The initial observation of increased prevalence of PFO in migraneurs came out in 1998 (1). Then subsequently several studies looked specifically for the prevalence of PFO in Migraneurs. Anzola and colleagues performed a case control study including 113 consecutive patients with migraine with aura, 53 patients with migraine without aura and 25 ages matched no migraine subjects. The presence of PFO was assessed indirectly by using transcranial Doppler sonography with IV. Injection of agitated saline. The prevalence of PFO was 48% in patients with migraine with aura, 23% in patients with migraine without aura and 20% in controls. The difference between migraine with aura and migraine without aura was significant (odds ratio=3.13) as well as between migraine with aura and control group (odds ratio=3.66) (19).

Schwedt et al. (2008) performed a systematic review of 18 out of 134 identified articles to examine the prevalence of migraine in patients with PFO. The results demonstrated that people with migraine with aura are more likely to have a PFO than people with migraine without aura or healthy controls (20). Migraine with aura not related with diving occurred significantly more frequently in patients with large right to left shunt which was present at rest (38 of 80, 47.5%), compared with patients who had a smaller shunt (four of 40, 10%) or with patients with no shunt at all (11 of 80, 13.8%). The prevalence of migraine without aura was similar in all groups. Authors concluded that migraine with aura was associated with presence or absence of PFO but also with the shunt size (21).

McCandless et al (2011) conducted pediatric study involved a population consisted of 109 children with migraine; 38 (35%) with aura and 71 (65%) without aura. The overall PFO prevalence was 35%, similar to the general population (35% vs. 25%; P = .13). However, compared with the general population (25%), the PFO prevalence was significantly greater in subjects with aura (50%, P = .0004) but similar in those without aura (27%, P = .73). Atrial shunt size was not associated with the presence or absence of aura. Their conclusion was that Children with migraine with aura have a significantly higher prevalence of PFO compared with those without aura or the general population. These data suggest that PFO may contribute to the pathogenesis of migraine with aura in children and have implications for clinical decision making (22).

A meta analysis of 7 studies in adult population with migraine headache and aura showed association of PFO in this particular population ranging from 41- 62% (composite of 56% by meta-analysis) (23-29).

On the other hand; NOMAS study (30) involved screening of population from Northern Manhattan area showed no significant association of PFO with Migraine headache population. This study has several limitations though. It included only non-stroke patients who are older than 39 years, they used Trans thoracic Echocardiography for the screen of PFO with no Trans Cranial Doppler evaluation of the bubble study and they depended on self-reporting headache with obvious recall bias.

Table one summarized the major studies of PFO association with Migraine headache. It is clear from all previously mentioned studies that Migraine with Aura has higher association of PFO compared to migraine without aura. Both (with and without aura) has higher prevalence of PFO compared to general population please see Table 1.

Study	PFO Method	Migraine With Aura, n/N (%)	Migraine Without Aura, n/N (%)
Del Sette et al	TCD	18/44 (41)	NA
Anzola et al	TCD	54/113 (48)	12/53 (23)
Schwerzmann et al	TEE	44/93 (47)	NA
Dalla Volta et al	TCD	161/260 (62)	12/74 (16)
Carod-Artal et al	TCD	25/48 (52)	32/93 (34)
Domitrz et al	TCD	33/61 (54)	15/60 (25)
NOMAS	TTE	26/140 (19)	4/38 (11)

TCD indicates transcranial Doppler; TEE, transesophageal echocardiography.

Table 1. Prevalence of PFO Among Subjects With Migraine Selected From the Literature

The prevailing hypothesis regarding the pathogenesis of migraine is an inherited excitability of certain brain networks that, when triggered by particular endogenous or exogenous factors, leads to a cascade of events that result in head pain. The presence of PFO might trigger this process by allowing substances or metabolites to pass from the hepatic or portal circulation to the carotids circulation. Migraneurs have increased platelet activation and aggregation in response to serotonin. Normally serotonin is metabolized by lung mono amino oxidase (MAO), but if blood is shunted through a PFO and avoids the pulmonary circulation it has been postulated that this can trigger migraine onset and precipitate aura (31). Another mechanism could possibly be transient hypoxemia caused by the PFO, causing subclinical infarcts in the brain, leading to irritation and propensity for migraines. Naqvi et al. report different manifestations of PFO including resting and stress hypoxemia related to left to right shunting across a PFO in the absence of pulmonary hypertension (32).

4. Results of studies of PFO closure to relief migraine headaches

Initial observation from studies involves Stroke prevention by PFO device-closure, showed patients with Migraine headaches improve after the procedures (34-38).

Recently Wahl et al (2010) reported a large cohort of Migraneurs (150 patients 96 of them had aura) who underwent closure of PFO for stroke prevention. Of those 34% showed complete resolution of the headache and 48% showed significant improvement of their headaches, making total of 82% of the migraneurs benefited from the closure. The presence of aura was associated with higher improvement in their study population. Still they showed improvement in non-aura migraneurs.

Daniela Trabattoni reviewed 305 patients who underwent closure of their PFO for stroke prevention, 77 of them have migraine headache (~55% are female). Follow up of these migraine patients at 3 months showed complete cessation of headache in 46% of the patients and 40% had improvement of their headache intensity score (total improvement of 86% of the patients). They found maintenance of these results up to 5 years of follow up (44).

After these initial observations of improved migraine headache in the patients who underwent prevention of stroke by device-closure of their PFO (table 2), then several studies were conducted primarily for Migraine headaches relief.

Author, year (Ref.)	N of pts	Patients with migraine	Pts with migraine and aura	Pts with migraine without aura	Age migraine-pts	Sex (F/M) MH- pts	Indications for defect closure	Defect type	Devices used
Anzola, 2006 [16]	77	77 (100%)	54 (70%)	23 (30%)	Between 36 ± 11 and 40 ± 12 (see text)	58/19	Stroke pts and no stroke pts with MH (see text)	PFO	NA
Morandi, 2003 [18]	17	17 (100%)	8 (47%)	9 (53%)	48 ± 11	12/5	Stroke	PFO	Amplatzer
Reisman, 2005 [19]	162	50 (31%)	38 (76%)	12 (24%)	47 ± 12	38/12	Stroke	PFO	Amplatzer = 11 pts CardioSeal: 151 pts
Post, 2004 [22]	66	26 (39%)	12 (46%)	14 (54%)	55 ± 10	9/17	Stroke and peripheral embolism	PFO	NA
Schwerzmann, 2004 [23]	215	48 (22%)	37 (77 %)	11 (23 %)	49 ± 11 MHA 49 ± 12 MHnoA	31/17	Stroke and decompression illness	PFO	NA
Giardini, 2006 [24]	131	35 (27%)	35 (100 %)	0 (0%)	45 ± 13	10/25	Stroke	PFO	Amplatzer = 71 pts CardioSeal = 52 pts Helex = 8 pts
Slavin, 2007 [25]	131	50 (42%)	40 (80%)	10 (20%)	45.7 ± 11.5	36/14	Stroke	PFO	Amplatzer 101 pts CardioSeal = 30 pts
Dubiel, 2008 [28]	191	46 (24%)	24 (52%)	22 (48%)	44 ± 13.5	35/11	Stroke	PFO	Amplatzer = 38 pts Cardio-SEAL/Starflex = 8 pts
MIST, 2008 [29]	147	74 (100%)	74 (100%)	0 (%)	44.6 ± 10.6	12/62	Migraine with aura	PFO	Starflex = 74 pts
Jesurum, 2008 [30]	77	77 (100%)	55 (71%)	22 (29%)	47 ± 12 MHA 46 ± 10 MhnoA	57/20	Stroke or paradoxical embolism	PFO	CardioSeal = 67 pts Amplatzer = 10 pts
Luermans, 2008 [31]	92	24 (28,6%)	10 (42%)	14 (58%)	51.6 ± 12.3	9/15	Stroke or paradoxical embolism	PFO	Amplatzer = 7 pts CardioSeal/Star-flex = 42 pts Cardiastar = 38 pts Helex = 2 pts
Total	1,306	524 (40%)	387 (74%)	137 (26%)					

Table 2. Meta Analysis of 11 studies reported by Gianfranco Butera et al (40)

Luciane Piazza et al. evaluated 42 patients with migraine headache (28 with aura and 14 without aura) after PFO closure for the migraine headache as a primary reason. After 6 months follow up they found complete resolution of the migraine in 26%, and significant improvement in 52% of the study group. Interestingly they found patients improvement (total 78%) regardless of the presence of aura history. Multiple logistic regression analysis showed that the improvement in migraine with aura and migraine without aura was independent of migraine type, sex, age, cerebrovascular risk factors and cerebrovascular events, type of cardiac defect, and thrombophilic conditions (41).

Another study by Andreas Wahl and his group was conducted on 17 patients with Migraine headache underwent closure of the PFO primarily for the headache reason (no stroke). They found total improvement in 71% of their patients with complete resolution of the headache in 26%. Their follow up was up to 30 months. They found slightly higher improvement in patients with aura (42).

Gianluca Rigatelli et al. conducted prospective study on 34 patients with Migraine headache (22 females and 12 male) and underwent closure of the atrial defect by one of two devices (Amplatz cribriform, AGA PFO device or Premere Occlusion System). They found about 55% of their study group have moderate to large atrial septal aneurysm. After a median of 9 months follow up period they have significant improvement in all the patients with 20 patients stopped completely their anti headache medications and the rest have improvement with less number of their medications (43).

The only randomized prospective study with patients blinded for PFO closure conducted for migraine headache is MIST trial. They included about 147 patients randomized for device closure or Sham procedure (patients will have general anesthesia with incision in the groin without device implantation). The study had an ambitious primary end point which was complete cessation of Migraine headache in 40% of the patients who receive PFO device closure. They chose STARFlex® and they have much higher rate of complications in their study (~12%) compared to other PFO device studies. They showed in 6 months no statistical difference between the two groups in complete cessation of Migraine headache. *Post-hoc* analysis revealed that, when two extreme outliers were removed, a significant reduction in the median total headache days was observed in patients assigned to PFO closure ($P = 0.027$). A number of methodological reasons could explain why the primary end point of the MisT trial was not achieved. First, this ambitious primary end point, presumably selected to justify the risks of an interventional procedure, was so strict as to be unrealistic, and was arguably less clinically relevant than a quantifiable reduction in headache days. Although the path physiology of migraine is not fully elucidated, the probable multifactorial nature of migraine triggers means that correction of one potential trigger is unlikely to result in headache cure. Second, the patients for whom migraine improvement was previously reported had PFO closure for either cryptogenic stroke or decompression illness. However, such patients were specifically excluded from the MIST trial. The amount of residual shunt in MIST trial was extremely high (~35%) in 6 months follow up probably due to inherent device limitations used in the study. Other potential confounding factors include the 'hangover effect' of antiplatelet therapy and the difficulty of distinguishing between cardiac-level and pulmonary-level shunt when using transthoracic echocardiography (TTE). nonetheless, as the first randomized, controlled trial of its kind, the MIST trial has pioneered a robust study design for PFO closure trials and raised questions to be addressed in future studies.

In Summery: The association of migraine headache with Patent Foramen Ovale is higher than normal population (more than double) by most of the studies. Trans Cranial Doppler has higher sensitivity than Echo (TTE, TEE or ICE) in detecting the right to left shunt across the atrial septum. Because of the anatomical orientation of the Inferior Vena Cava towards the Foramen Ovale, injection of bubble contrast in lower limbs veins might be higher sensitive than injection in upper limbs veins. Whether the PFO/Migraine association means also a causation relationship: a question still needs more definite answer. Most of the studies (from stroke studies and primary studies for Migraine relief) are pointing towards the causation relationship. Although the only randomized prospective study in the literature failed to show a definite answer, several confounding factors (as mentioned above in the text) can explain the negativity of this study. Most of the studies showed higher response and benefit to patients suffer from Migraine with aura compared to others.

5. References

[1] Del Sette M, Angeli S, Leandri M, Ferriero G, Bruzzone GL, Finocchi C, Gandolfo C. Migraine with aura and right-to-left shunt on transcranial Doppler: a case control study. *Cerebrovasc Dis.* 1998;8:327–330.

[2] Hagen PT, Scholz DG, Edwards WD. Incidence and size of patent foramen ovale during the first 10 decades of life: an autopsy study of 965 normal hearts. *Mayo Clin Proc.* 1984;59:17–20.

[3] Di Tullio MR, Sacco RL, Sciacca RR, Jin Z, Homma S. Patent foramen ovale and the risk of ischemic stroke in a multiethnic population. *J Am Coll Cardiol.* 2007;49:797- 802.

[4] Meissner I, Whisnant JP, Khanderia BK, Spittell PC, O'Fallon WM, Pascoe RD, Enriquez-Sarano M, Seward JB, Covalt JL, Sicks JD, Wiebers DO. Prevalence of potential risk factors for stroke assessed by transesophageal echocardiography and carotid ultrasonography: the SPARC study Stroke Prevention: Assessment of Risk in a Community. *Mayo Clin Proc.* 1999;74:862- 869.

[5] Choong, C. K. *et al.* Life-threatening impending paradoxical embolus caught "red-handed": successful management by multidisciplinary team approach. *J. Thorac. Cardiovasc. Surg.* 136, 527–528 (2008).

[6] Kim, R. J. & Girardi, L. N. "Lots of clots": multiple thromboemboli including a huge paradoxical embolus in a 29-year old man. *Int. J. Cardiol.* 129, e50–e52 (2008).

[7] Madani, H. & Ransom, P. A. Paradoxical embolus illustrating speed of action of recombinant tissue plasminogen activator in massive pulmonary embolism. *Emerg. Med. J.* 24, 441 (2007).

[8] Ahmed, S., Sadiq, A., Siddiqui, A. K., Borgen, E. & Mattana, J. Paradoxical arterial emboli causing acute limb ischemia in a patient with essential thrombocytosis. *Am. J. Med. Sci.* 326, 156–158 (2003).

[9] Lipton RB, Bigal ME, Diamond M, Freitag F, Reed ML, Stewart WF. Migraine prevalence, disease burden, and the need for preventative therapy. Neurology 2007;68:343–9.

[10] Stovner LJ, Hagen K, Jensen R, et al. The global burden of headache: a documentation of headache prevalence and disability worldwide. Cephalalgia 2007;27:193–210.

[11] Goadsby PJ, Lipton RB, Ferrari MD. Migraine: current understanding and treatment. *N Engl J Med.* 2002;346:257–270.

[12] Wilmshurst PT, Pearson MJ, Nightingale S, Walsh KP, Morrison WL. Inheritance of persistent foramen ovale and atrial septal defects and the relation to familial migraine with aura. *Heart*. 2004;90:1315–1320.

[13] Del Sette M, Angeli S, Leandri M, Ferriero G, Bruzzone GL, Finocchi C, Gandolfo C. Migraine with aura and right-to-left shunt on transcranial Doppler: a case control study. *Cerebrovasc Dis*. 1998;8:327–330.

[14] Charles A. Advances in the basic and clinical science of migraine. Ann Neurol 2009;65:491- 8.

[15] Wilmshurst PT, Pearson MJ, Nightingale S, et al. Inheritance of persistent foramen ovale and atrial septal defects and the relation to familial migraine with aura. Heart 2004;90:1315-20.

[16] Lipton RB, Bigal ME, Diamond M, Freitag F, Reed ML, Stewart WF. Migraine prevalence, disease burden, and the need for preventative therapy. Neurology 2007;68:343–9.

[17] Stovner LJ, Hagen K, Jensen R, et al. The global burden of headache: a documentation of headache prevalence and disability worldwide. Cephalalgia 2007;27:193–210.

[18] Abu-Arefeh I, Russell G. Prevalence of headache and migraine in schoolchildren. BMJ 1994;309:765-9.

[19] Anzola GP, Frisoni GB, Morandi E, et al. Shunt associated migraine responds favorably to atrial septal repair: a case control study. Stroke 2006;37:430–4.

[20] Schwedt TJ, Demaerschalk BM, Dodick DW. Patent foramen ovale and migraine: a quantitative systematic review. Cephalalgia 2008;28:531–40.

[21] Wilmshurst PT, Nightingale S, Walsh KP, et al. Effect on migraine of closure of cardiac right-to-left shunts to prevent recurrence of decompression illness or stroke or for haemodynamic reasons. Lancet 2000;356:1648–51.

[22] Rachel T. McCandless, MD, Cammon B. Arrington, MD, Douglas C. Nielsen, James F. Bale, Jr., MD, and L. LuAnn Minich, MD. Patent Foramen Ovale in Children with Migraine Headaches. J Pediatr 2011;159:243-7.

[23] Agmon Y, Khandheria BK, Meissner I, Gentile F, Sicks JD, O'FallonWM, et al. Comparison of frequency of patent foramen ovale by transesophageal echocardiography in patients with cerebral ischemic events versus in subjects in the general population. Am J Cardiol 2001;88:330-2..

[24] Del Sette M, Angeli S, Leandri M, Ferriero G, Bruzzone GL, Finocchi C, Gandolfo C. Migraine with aura and right-to-left shunt on transcranial Doppler: a case-control study. Cerebrovasc Dis 1998;8:327-30.

[25] Anzola GP, Magoni M, Guindani M, Rozzini L, Dalla Volta G. Potential source of cerebral embolism in migraine with aura: a transcranial Doppler study. Neurology 1999;52:1622-5.

[26] Domitrz I, Mieszkowski J, Kaminska A. Relationship between migraine and patent foramen ovale: a study of 121 patients with migraine. Headache 2007;47:1311-8.

[27] Schwerzmann M, Nedeltchev K, Lagger F, Mattle HP, Windecker S, Meier B, Seiler C. Prevalence and size of directly detected patent foramen ovale in migraine with aura. Neurology 2005;65:1415-8.

[28] Schwerzmann M, Nedeltchev K, Meier B. Patent foramen ovale closure: a new therapy for migraine. Catheter Cardiovasc Interv 2007;69:277-84.

[29] Garg P, Servoss SJ, Wu JC, Bajwa ZH, Selim MH, Dineen A, et al. Lack of association between migraine headache and patent foramen ovale: results of a case-control study. Circulation 2010;121:1406-12.

[30] Tatjana Rundek, Mitchell S.V. Elkind, Marco R. Di Tullio, Emmanuel Carrera, Zhezhen Jin, Ralph L. Sacco and Shunichi Homma. Northern Manhattan Study (NOMAS) Patent Foramen Ovale and Migraine : A Cross-Sectional Study From the Northern Manhattan Study (NOMAS). *Circulation* 2008, 118:1419-1424

[31] Zeller JA, Frahm K, Baron R, et al: Platelet-Leukocyte Interaction and Platelet Activation in Migraine: A link to ischemic stroke? *J Neurol Neurosurg Psychiatry* 2004;75:984–987.

[32] Naqvi T, Rafie R, Daneshvar S: Potential Faces of Patent Foramen Ovale. *Echocardiogr* 2010;27:897–907.

[33] Wilmshurst PT, Nightingale S, Walsh KP, et al. Effect on migraine of closure of cardiac right-to-left shunts to prevent recurrence of decompression illness or stroke or for haemodynamic reasons. Lancet 2000;356:1648-51.

[34] Schwerzmann M, Wiher S, Nedeltchev K, et al. Percutaneous closure of patent foramen ovale reduces the frequency of migraine attacks. Neurology 2004;62:1399-401.

[35] Post MC, Thijs V, Herroelen L, et al. Closure of a patent foramen ovale is associated with a decrease in prevalence of migraine. Neurology 2004;62:1439-40.

[36] Azarbal B, Tobis J, Suh W, et al. Association of interatrial shunts and migraine headaches: impact of transcatheter closure. J Am Coll Cardiol 2005;45:489-92.

[37] Reisman M, Christofferson RD, Jesurum J, et al. Migraine headache relief after transcatheter closure of patent foramen ovale. J Am Coll Cardiol 2005;45:493-5.

[38] Giardini A, Donti A, Formigari R, et al. Transcatheter patent foramen ovale closure mitigates aura migraine headaches abolishing spontaneous right-to-left shunting. Am Heart J 2006;151:922

[39] Andreas Wahl, Fabien Praz, Tony Tai, Oliver Findling, Nazan Walpoth, Krassen Nedeltchev, Markus Schwerzmann, Stephan Windecker, Heinrich P Mattle, Bernhard Meier. Improvement of migraine headaches after percutaneous closure of patent foramen ovale for secondary prevention of paradoxical embolism. Heart 2010; 96:967-973.

[40] Gianfranco Butera, Giuseppe G. L. Biondi-Zoccai, Mario Carminati, Luigi Caputi, Susanna Usai, Gennaro Bussone, Giovanni Meola, Angelica Bibiana Delogu, Imad Sheiban and Giuseppe Sangiorgi. Systematic Review and Meta-Analysis of Currently Available Clinical Evidence on Migraine and Patent Foramen Ovale Percutaneous Closure: Much Ado About Nothing? Catheterization and Cardiovascular Interventions 75:494–504 (2010)

[41] Massimo Chessa, Chiara Colombo, Gianfranco Butera, Diana Negura, Luciane Piazza, Leonardo Varotto, Claudio Bussadori, Vlasta Fesslova, Giovanni Meola and Mario Carminati. Is it too early to recommend patent foramen ovale closure for all patients who suffer from migraine? A single-centre study. Journal of Cardiovascular Medicine 2009, 10:401–405

[42] Andreas Wahl, Fabien Praz, Oliver Findling, Krassen Nedeltchev, Markus Schwerzmann, Tony Tai, Stephan Windecker, Heinrich P. Mattle, and Bernhard Meier. Percutaneous Closure of Patent Foramen Ovale for Migraine Headaches Refractory to Medical Treatment. Catheterization and Cardiovascular Interventions 74:124–129 (2009)

[43] Gianluca Rigatelli, Paolo Cardaioli, Fabio Dell'Avvocataa, Massimo Giordan, Gabriele Braggion, Mauro Chinaglia, Loris Roncon. Transcatheter patent foramen ovale closure is effective in reducing migraine independently from specific interatrial septum anatomy and closure devices design. Cardiovascular Revascularization Medicine 11 (2010) 29–33

[44] Daniela Trabattoni, Franco Fabbiocchi, Piero Montorsi, Stefano Galli, Giovanni Teruzzi, Luca Grancini, Pamela Gatto, and Antonio L. Bartorelli. Sustained Long-Term Benefit of Patent Foramen Ovale Closure on Migraine. Catheterization and Cardiovascular Interventions 77:570–574 (2011)

11

Transcatheter Occlusion of Atrial Septal Defects for Prevention of Recurrence of Paradoxical Embolism

Nicoleta Daraban, Manuel Reyes and Richard W. Smalling
University of Texas Health Science Center at Houston, Texas, USA

1. Introduction

Stroke is the third most common cause of death in the United States. Stroke also results in substantial health-care expenditures with an estimated lifetime cost from an ischemic stroke of $140,000 per patient (Rosamond K, 2007). Each year, approximately 795,000 people experience a new or recurrent stroke, of which an estimated 610,000 are first attacks. Mortality data from 2006 indicates stroke accounted for approximately 1 of every 18 deaths in the United States. On average, every 40 seconds, someone in the United States has a stroke (Heart Disease and Stroke Statistics, AHA 2009).

Cryptogenic infarction has had a predominant status among the causes of ischemic strokes, originally demonstrated in the Stroke Data Bank. Sacco and Mohr reported a 40% incidence of cryptogenic stroke in their population (Sacco, Ellenberg, Mohr et al., 1989). A cryptogenic infarction does not have a defined cause despite a complete work-up. It differs from infarction of undetermined causes, which may involve overlapping causes or an incomplete investigation.

Numerous studies have established a higher prevalence of patent foramen ovale (PFO) or atrial septal defect (ASD) in patients with cryptogenic stroke when compared to patients with stroke of determined cause despite correction for recognized stroke risk factors. This relationship has perpetuated the paradoxical embolism theory as a likely stroke mechanism in this patient population (Lechat 1988, Webster 1988, DeBelder 1992, DiTullio 1992).

Emboli leading to stroke can originate either in the systemic arterial circulation or in the systemic venous circulation (paradoxical embolism). A paradoxical embolus originates in the systemic venous circulation and enters the systemic arterial circulation through a PFO, ASD, ventricular septal defect (VSD), or extracardiac communication such as a pulmonary arteriovenous malformation (AVM).

Therapeutic measures for secondary prevention in this patient population can encompass medical treatment or surgical/percutaneous closure of the patent foramen ovale or atrial septal defect as well as coil embolization of pulmonary arteriovenous malformations.

Ongoing randomized clinical studies aim at comparing medical treatment versus closure of atrial septal defects to determine the most effective treatment strategy in this patient population (RESPECT PFO trial, CLOSURE I trial, Gore REDUCE Clinical Study "HLX 06-03).

Embryology of atrial septal defects

Patent Foramen Ovale

The foramen ovale is a pivotal feature during intrauterine life. The interatrial communication is necessary for the shunting of oxygenated blood from right atrium to left atrium. Beginning at four weeks of pregnancy the primordial atrial septum divides into right and left sides by formation and fusion of two septa: the septum primum and septum secundum. The interatrial septum primum on the left side and interatrial septum secundum on the right side maintain a central opening after having grown from the periphery to the center. This perforation is positioned caudally in the septum secundum and cranially in the septum primum, forming a slit valve that opens when right atrial pressure exceeds the left atrial pressure. The oxygenated blood from the umbilical vein entering through the inferior vena cava from the bottom of the right atrium keeps this window open until after birth.

Postnatal physiologic changes

At birth, right heart pressure and pulmonary vascular resistance drop as pulmonary arterioles open in reaction to oxygen filling the alveoli. Left atrial pressure may also rise as the amount of the blood returning from the lung increases. Either or both of these mechanisms may cause flap closure against the septum secundum.

This fusion is complete by age two in about 75% of individuals, but persistent patency occurs in the other 25% (Hagen, Scholz & Edwards, 1984). The reasons PFOs fail to close are unknown, but it is currently assumed they are likely related to multifactorial inheritance.

Atrial Septal Defect

One of the most common adult congenital heart defects, an atrial septal defect (ASD) is a persistent communication between the atria. Much like a patent foramen ovale, an ASD arises from incomplete fusion of the septum primum and septum secundum.

There are several different types of ASDs (see Figure 1):

- Secundum ASD in the region of the fossa ovalis;
- Primum ASD, positioned inferiorly near the crux of the heart;
- Sinus venosus ASD, located superiorly near the superior vena caval entry or inferiorly near the inferior vena caval entry; and
- The uncommon coronary sinus septal defect, which causes shunting into the left atrium via a communication in the superior aspect of the coronary sinus, posterior to the left atrium.

PFO Anatomy and Associated Anomalies

The autopsy-derived prevalence of PFO is 27% with decreasing prevalence at each decade of life. The PFO is a residual, oblique, slit-shaped defect resembling a tunnel. In adults, the persistent patent foramen ovale slit width ranges from 1 to 19 mm (mean 4.9 mm)

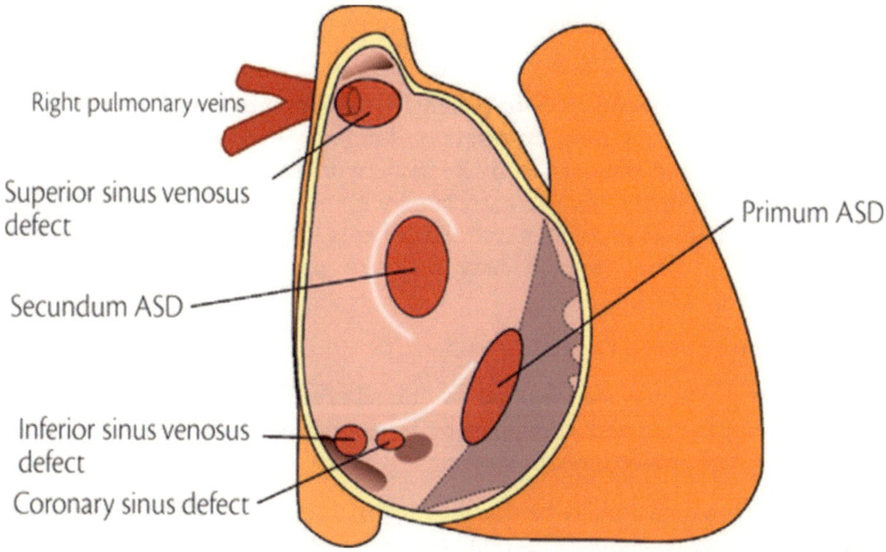

Fig. 1. Types of atrial septal defects. The **European Association of Echocardiography Textbook.**

(Hagen, Scholz & Edwards, 1984). The PFO size increases with age, reflecting size-based selection over time where larger PFOs remain patent and smaller defects close. Greater PFO size increases the risk of paradoxical embolism (Steiner, DiTullio, Rundek et al., 1998). Heterogeneity of size and morphology are pertinent to interventional device closure selection.

The histopathology of the PFO has not been thoroughly addressed in literature, although it is a point of increasing importance as percutaneous closure technologies must interact with these tissues at cellular level. The muscular atrial wall consists of endocardium having endothelium and thick subendothelial layers of connective tissue rich in collagen and elastin. A thicker myocardium lies beneath these structures, with loosely arranged musculature.

PFOs are associated with several anatomic anomalies, most commonly with atrial septal aneurysms (ASA) and Chiari networks.

An ASA represents an aneurysmal dilatation of a part or all of the septum primum, protruding into either atrium. The ASA is defined as phasic septal excursion of at least 10 mm during the cardiorespiratory cycle. M-mode transesophageal echocardiography (TEE) or intracardiac echocardiography is essential for precisely measuring septal excursion of the ASA. A persistent ASA can be isolated finding but generally is associated with other ASDs or a PFO. Fenestrated ASA may present with the clinical findings of an ASD with a significant left to right shunt, especially if there are multiple defects.

The Chiari network is a remnant of the right valve of the sinus venosus, and its role is poorly understood. It originates from a region of the Eustachian and Thebesian valves with attachment to the upper wall of the right atrium or atrial septum. The Eustachian valve is common but it should be distinguished from Chiari networks because it does not attach to the upper wall of the right atrium or atrial septum, although it may be mobile and fenestrated.

In a study of 1436 adult patients, 83% of patients were found to have both Chiari networks and a PFO, suggesting a strong association. Large right-to-left shunting was found significantly more often in patients with Chiari networks than in controls (55% vs. 12%). This study also found Chiari networks associated with ASAs in 24% of patients. The Chiari network is more common in cryptogenic stroke patients than in patients evaluated for other indications (4.6% vs. 0.5%), and it may facilitate paradoxical embolism (Schneider, Hofmann, Justen et al., 1995).

Diagnosis of Patent Foramen Ovale

A patent foramen ovale may be detected by transthoracic echocardiography (TTE), TEE, transcranial Doppler (TCD), and sometimes by transmitral Doppler. These techniques were compared in studies of proven embolic stroke.

Although the PFO can occasionally be documented in adults with a TTE, the result is rarely unequivocal. TEE, rather than TTE, remains the diagnosis method of choice, due to increased sensitivity.

PFO detection can be augmented by cough or releasing of a sustained Valsalva maneuver, while injecting an aerated colloidal solution into the systemic venous circulation (the bubble test, agitated saline, or contrast study). These maneuvers open the foramen when the right atrium fills with blood from the abdomen, while the left atrium volume is depleted before blood coming through the pulmonary veins, and thus the right atrial pressure exceeds the left atrial pressure.

The Valsalva maneuver is now considered necessary to find right-to-left shunts when performing echocardiography of any type, with or without contrast injection. The physical hole in the atrial wall may not be imaged, but detecting its shunt clearly improves sensitivity and specificity.

TCD is comparable to contrast TEE for detecting PFO-related right-to-left shunts echocardiography and is easy to perform at bedside (Sloan, Alexandrov, Tegeler et al., 2004). TCD has recently been augmented by power M-Mode, a technology that allows power display with Doppler velocity and velocity signals over selectable depth ranges along the transducer beam. TCD M-mode enhances sensitivity to contrast bubble emboli over single-gated examination (Spencer, Moehring, Jesurum et al., 2004; Moehring & Spencer, 2002).

Rationale for PFO and ASD treatment in patients with paradoxical embolism

As mentioned before, approximately 40% of ischemic strokes have no clear etiology (i.e., cryptogenic strokes). Treatment of this particular type of stroke could have a significant impact on decreasing the stroke burden in the general population.

One study of 60 adults under 55 years of age with ischemic stroke compared contrast echocardiographic examinations with 100 normal subjects. PFO prevalence was significantly higher in the stroke group than in controls (40% vs. 10%). PFO was found in 26 stroke patients with no other identifiable cause, and the study concluded that the PFO-induced paradoxical embolism is a cause of stroke (Lechat, Mas, Lascault et al., 1988).

The PFO-ASA Study supports these findings, where 46% of young cryptogenic stroke patients had PFO (Lamy, Giannesini, Zuber et al., 2002).

Cramer et al. evaluated young stroke patients (18 to 60 years old) early after stroke using magnetic resonance imaging venography (Cramer, Rordorf, Maki, et al., 2004). Pelvic deep venous thrombosis was increased in the cryptogenic stroke population compared to controls (20% vs. 4%). The cryptogenic stroke group was significantly younger (42 vs. 49 years) with fewer risk factors for atherosclerosis, such as hypertension and smoking. PFO prevalence was significantly higher in the cryptogenic stroke group than in controls (59% vs. 19%).

A prospective study of 598 patients (ages 18 to 55 years) presenting with cryptogenic stroke showed that 36% had PFO, 1.7% had ASA and 8.5% had both abnormalities. Patients with both PFO and ASA who have had a stroke, are thus at higher risk for recurrent stroke, and preventive strategies other than aspirin should be considered (Mas, Arquizan, Lamy et al., 2001).

Decompression illness in divers is another PFO-associated clinical syndrome. Decompression syndrome (DCS) is categorized in type I and type II. Type I DCS is composed of localized joint pain, musculoskeletal pain, and/or skin rash, and type II DCS consists of neurologic symptoms (limb tingling, paresthesias, severe headache with mental confusion, paraplegia, loss of consciousness, audio vestibular symptoms, and dyspnea with chest pain). The PFO at rest is significantly associated with type II DCS.

In a seminal study, TCD ultrasonography detected a right-to-left shunt in all divers with multiple brain lesions suggesting the presence of a PFO (Knauth, Ries, Pohimann et al., 1997). A comparative investigation regarding brain lesions and the presence of a PFO in sport divers and non-diving controls showed that brain lesions were more common in individuals with a PFO, although divers had more brain lesions than non-divers, irrespective of the presence of a PFO (Schwerzmann, Seiler, Lipp et al., 2001). This has led some diving schools to recommend screening for the presence of a PFO for professional divers or avid amateurs.

The presumed mechanism of cerebral vascular events in patients with a patent foramen ovale or an atrial septal defect is a transient increase in right-sided pressure, which causes a right-to-left shunt. In this scenario, embolization into the left circulation may be produced from a small right-sided thrombus. It is possible, therefore, for paradoxical embolization to occur into other vascular beds such as the coronary artery system and cause an acute myocardial infarction. Few such cases of paradoxical coronary embolisms have been reported in the literature and the diagnosis was made by excluding other sources of coronary artery disease or embolization (Deborah, Gersony, Sang et al., 2001; Agostoni, Gasparini & Destro, 2004).

Medical versus surgical treatment of symptomatic atrial septal defects

Surgical closure has been demonstrated to be effective in the prevention of recurrent stroke (Mohr, Thompson, Lazar et al., 2001). However, due to the risks and expense of open-heart surgery, subjects are largely treated with oral anticoagulation and antiplatelet agents on an empirical basis.

The present empirical therapy of subjects with PFO and paradoxical embolism is far from ideal and it is uncertain whether anticoagulants such as warfarin and antiplatelet agents are effective as primary or secondary therapy in preventing stroke in patients with PFO.

The PFO in the Cryptogenic Stroke Study Investigators found no difference in primary end-points (recurrent stroke and death) between aspirin and warfarin treatment of PFO patients at two years (Bridges, Hellenbrand, Latson et al., 1992).

The Warfarin-Aspirin Recurrent Stroke Study was a prospective trial of 2206 patients with prior stroke (Homma, Sacco, Di Tullio et al., 2002). Patients were randomized to aspirin (325 mg/day) or warfarin (INR 1.4 to 2.8). After two years, the investigators concluded that there were no significant differences between aspirin and warfarin treatment for recurrent stroke or death. The incidence of recurrent stroke, transient ischemic attacks or death was 17.8 % per year in the warfarin group vs. 16% per year in the aspirin group. Patients with cryptogenic stroke showed no significant benefit in either treatment group.

The incidence of major hemorrhage (per 100 patients per year) was 2.2 in the warfarin group vs. 1.5 in the aspirin group. The authors note that higher target INRs (3.0-4.5) have been associated with excessive rates of major hemorrhage.

Bridges et al. found that despite 32 of 36 subjects being on warfarin therapy before device closure, the recurrence rate of stroke was 50% (Bridges, Hellenbrand, Latson et al., 1992). The appropriate duration of warfarin therapy is unknown and empirical and the incidence of major bleeding events ranges from 1.5 to 11% per year.

Catheter-Based PFO and ASD Closure

Some cerebrovascular events and other systemic arterial emboli, especially in young patients, are presumed to be due to paradoxical embolism through an atrial defect, most frequently a patent foramen ovale (PFO). Closure of such defects is an alternative to life-long anticoagulation.

Initial techniques of percutaneous ASD closure were documented with King's device in 1976 (Mills and King, 1976), Rashkind in the 1980's, and Sideris et al. in the 1990's (Mills and King 1976, Rashkind 1983, Sideris 1990).

Bridges et al. first proposed that PFO closure would reduce the incidence of recurrent strokes and demonstrated a statistically significant effect of PFO closure on a small group of high-risk patients (Bridges, Hellenbrand, Latson et al., 1992). Since then, numerous studies have shown that transcatheter PFO closure with current techniques is safe and seems to protect against recurrent strokes in this patient population (Kramer 2010, Krizanic 2010).

In the 1980s, the Rashkind occluder was introduced and revived the interest in the topic, focusing for the first time on the patent foramen ovale. The Rashkind Clamshell occluder was withdrawn from the market because of high incidence of stress fractures and breakage of arms. The clamshell device was modified by introducing an additional bend of the arms and reintroduced as the CardioSEAL device (1996). Subsequently the CardioSeal device was modified by introducing a self-centering mechanism and was renamed STARFlex (Nitinol Medical Technologies, Boston, Massachusetts, USA) (Kramer 2010).

In 1997, a new self-expanding Nitinol prosthesis was developed by Dr. Kurt Amplatz, which consists of two self-expandable round disks connected to each other with a short waist. Nitinol is a nickel-titanium alloy that has the property of resuming its initial shape when deployed (shape memory) (Krizanic 2010; Masura, Gavora et al., 1997). The Amplatzer device was approved by FDA in 2001 for ASD closure and has been widely used since. Several modifications of the Amplatzer device were introduced since its original design, such as the Amplatzer PFO occluder in 1999 and a cribriform device to occlude multiple or fenestrated ASDs.

In 2000, the CardioSEAL device (NMT Medical, Inc. - Boston, MA) and in 2002, the Amplatzer PFO Occluder (AGA Medical Corporation - Golden Valley, MN) became available for PFO closure in high-risk patients in the United States. Both devices were subsequently restricted to use in clinical trials evaluating device closure vs. medical therapy in patients with cryptogenic stroke and patent foramen ovale.

One of the devices used in current clinical trials for PFO closure is the Gore HELEX septal occluder. The HELEX device is made up of a single length nitinol wire covered by a thin membrane of expanded polytetrafluoroethylene (ePTFE). ePTFE (Gore-Tex) is a carbon and fluorine based synthetic polymer that is biologically inert and non-biodegradable in the body.

The configuration of the HELEX device consists of two flexible disks elongated around a central mandrel and delivered through a 9F sheath. The device was FDA approved in 2006 for ASD closure and is currently used in the REDUCE trial for PFO closure (The Gore REDUCE Clinical Study "HLX 06-03; Latson, Zahn & Wilson 2000).

A comprehensive review of the ASD closure devices has been addressed in several other chapters of this book and will not be further discussed.

The Amplatzer PFO occluder (AGA Medical Corporation - Golden Valley, MN) is currently the most used PFO closure device.

The Amplatzer occluder device consists of a nitinol double disk containing polyester fabric inside the two disks. A thin neck formed by the woven wires connects the two atrial disks. The neck is twisted around its long axis and hence is extendable. The device has to be screwed on to a pusher/puller cable and pulled into the introducer sheath. When pushed out of the sheath, it resumes its double-disk shape instantly. The whole process is fully reversible, as many times as required, up to the moment the device is unscrewed from the pusher/puller cable.

Three sizes of Amplatzer PFO closure devices are available and named after the diameter of the right sided disk- 18 mm, 25 mm, and 35 mm. The 18 mm PFO occluder comprises of two 18 mm disks and is meant for small PFOs with a stable septum primum. The 35 mm occluder is destined for large PFOs with atrial septal aneurysm and features a 35 mm disk on the right side and a 28 mm disk on the left side. It requires a 9 French sheath in contrast with the two smaller devices fitting through an 8 French sheath (Meier 2005).

The implantation can be performed with a single femoral venous puncture under fluoroscopy without echocardiographic guidance; however, in most institutions ICE is routinely performed to guide device placement both fluoroscopically and with ICE imaging (Image 1-5).

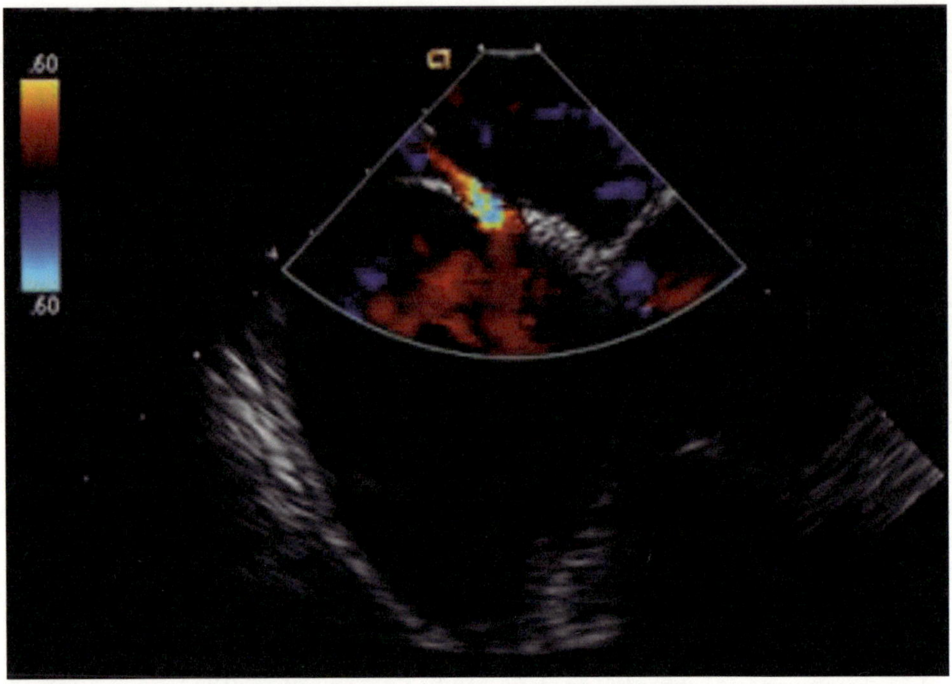

Image 1. ICE imaging of patent foramen ovale with Doppler ultrasound, showing blood flow in the tunnel between the septum primum and septum secundum.

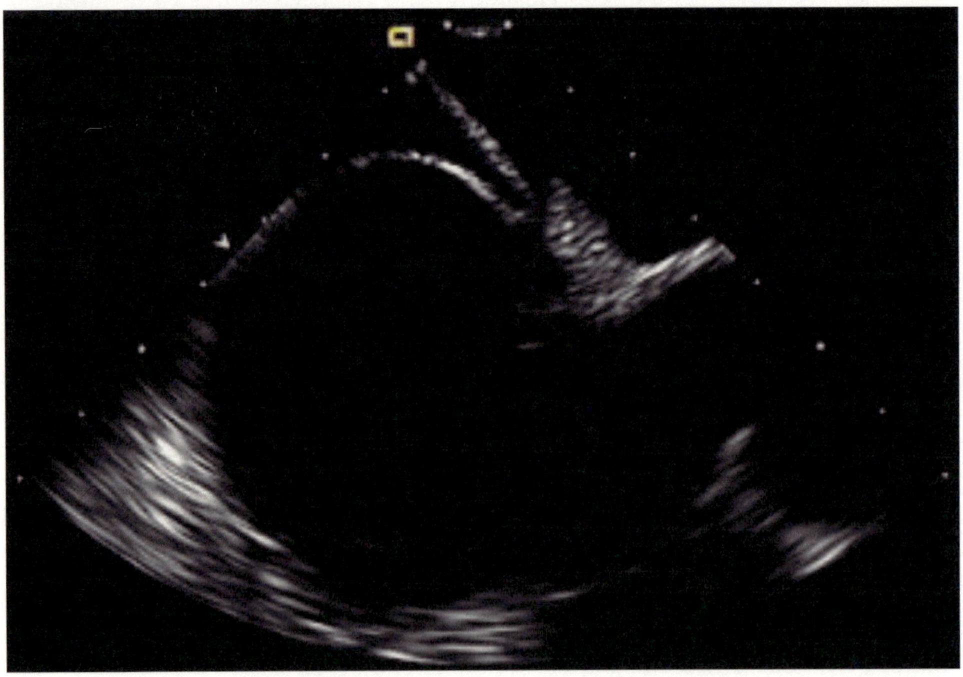

Image 2. ICE imaging of the diagnostic catheter engaging and crossing the tunnel between the septum primum and septum secundum.

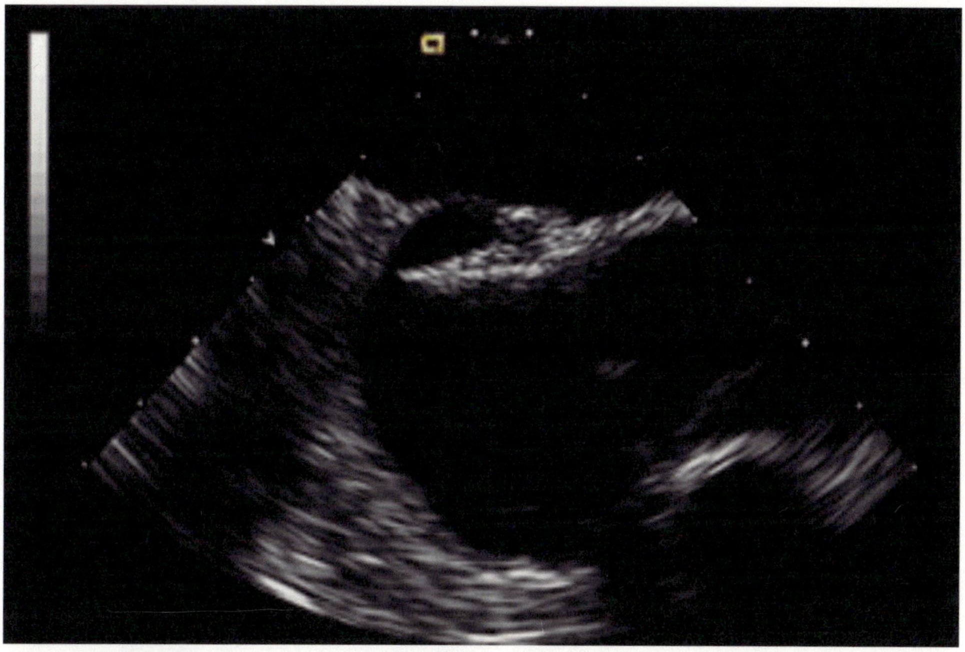

Image 3. Positioning of the left atrial disk under ICE guidance, against the left atrial side of the interatrial septum.

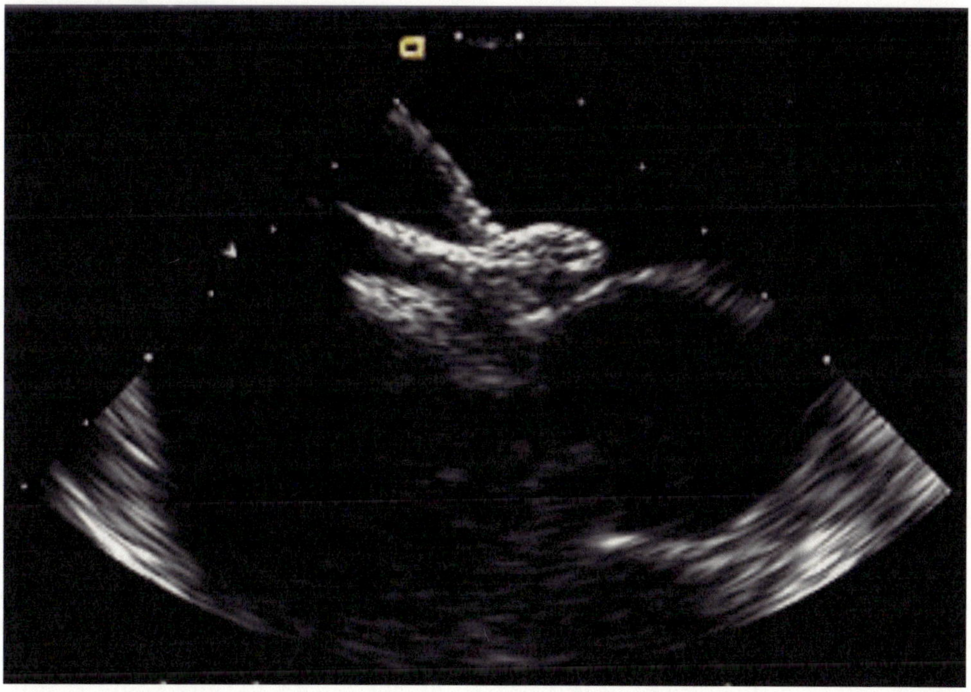

Image 4. Positioning of the right atrial disk under ICE guidance, on the right atrial side of the interatrial septum.

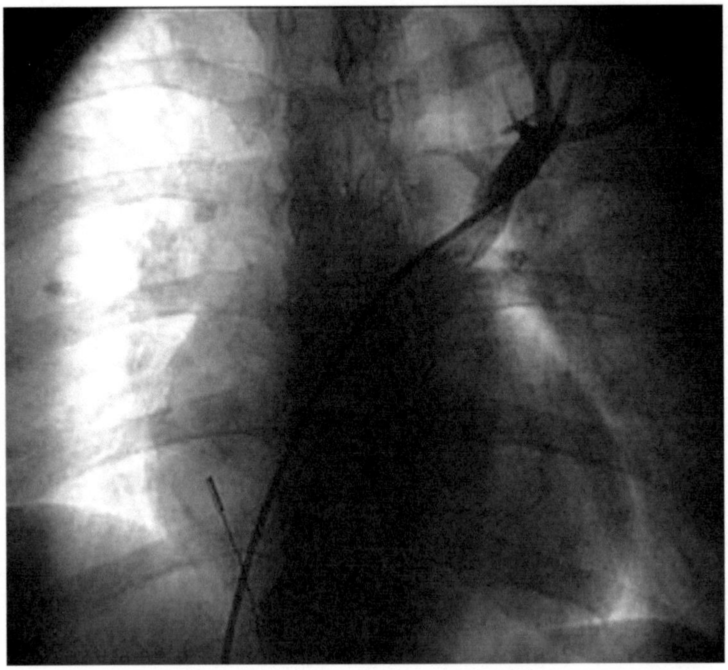

Image 5. Pulmonary vein angiogram through the Counard catheter, after crossing the PFO.

The PFO can be crossed by sliding along the septum primum, coming from the inferior vena cava with a wire or a curved catheter. A transvenous sheath (diameter 3 to 5 mm according to the device selected) is placed in to the left atrium (Image 3) and the position of the catheter is documented by pulmonary vein injection (Image 5). The left-sided disk is unfolded and pulled back against the septum, thereby pulling the septum primum against the septum secundum and closing the slit valve (Image 3). The right-sided disk is then deployed and the device released (Image 4). The perfect seat can be assessed before release by echocardiography or by hand-injected dye into the right atrium through the introducer (Image 6-9).

Follow-up treatment includes acetylsalicylic acid (80 to 300 mg) for a few months, with the addition of clopidogrel (75 mg) or warfarin (International Normalized Ratio 2.5 to 3.5) at some centers. Antibiotics during the interventions are commonplace, and prevention against endocarditis is recommended for a few months until the device is completely covered by tissue.

A follow-up transthoracic echocardiogram after a few months with no residual shunting signals the cessation of all treatment and controls.

Technical failures have become extremely rare (for example, inability to cannulate the PFO is less than 1%). Complications may include cardiac tamponade, symptomatic air embolism, loss of device, or puncture site problems.

Complete closure at follow-up can be expected in 90% to 95% of cases with the two US currently available devices. Some trivial residual shunt may be acceptable, albeit undesirable, as the device will act as a filter for particulate matter. Events have recurred in cases where

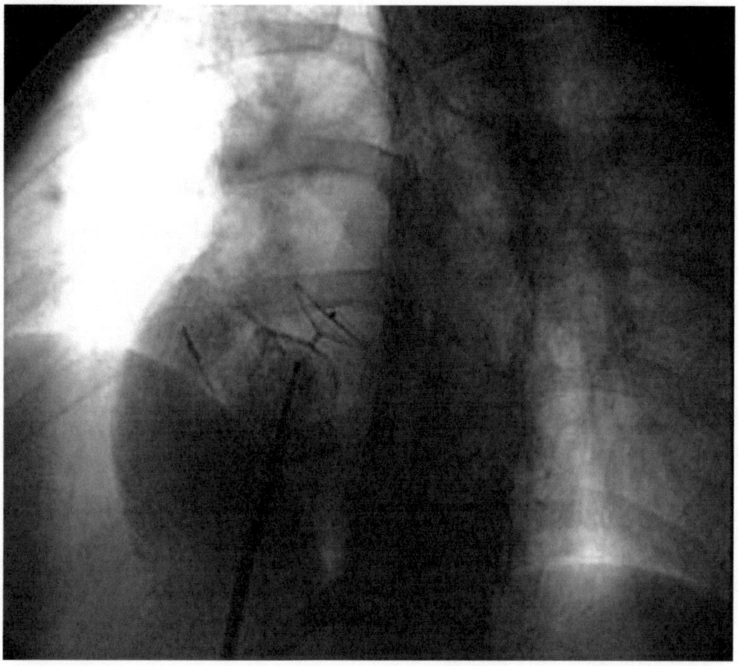

Image 6. Deployed PFO occluder under fluoroscopy, before the retrieval of the delivery catheter.

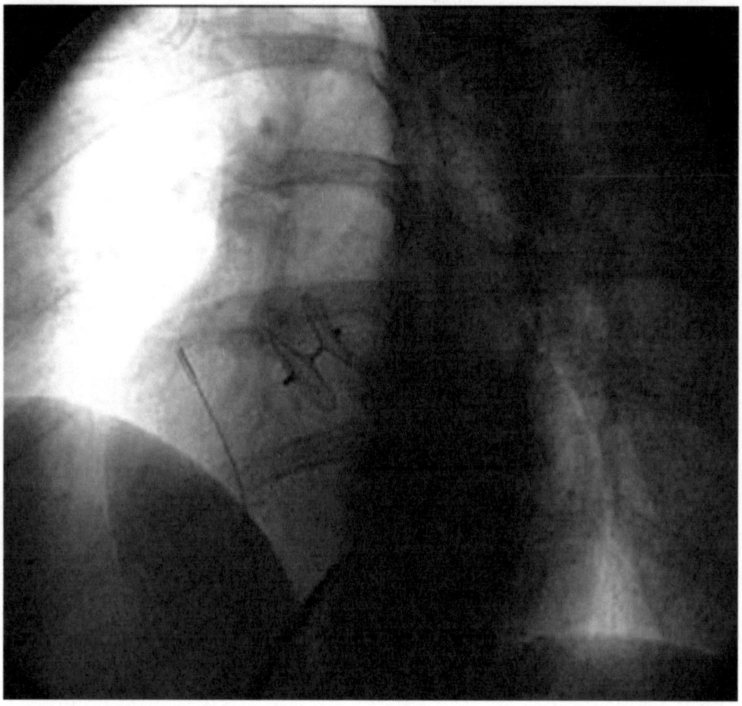

Image 7. Fully deployed PFO occluder under fluoroscopy.

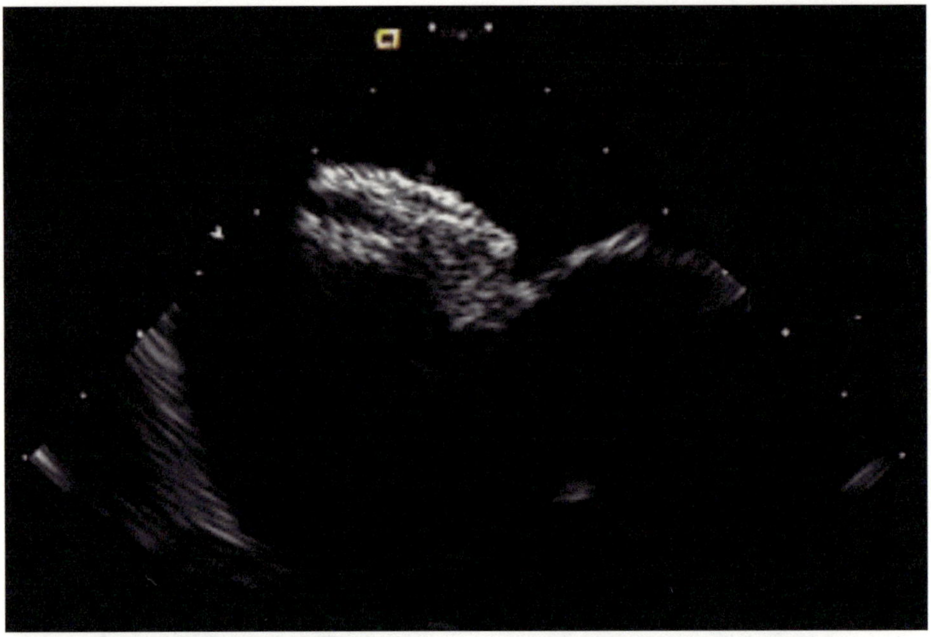

Image 8. Deployed PFO occluder under ICE imaging.

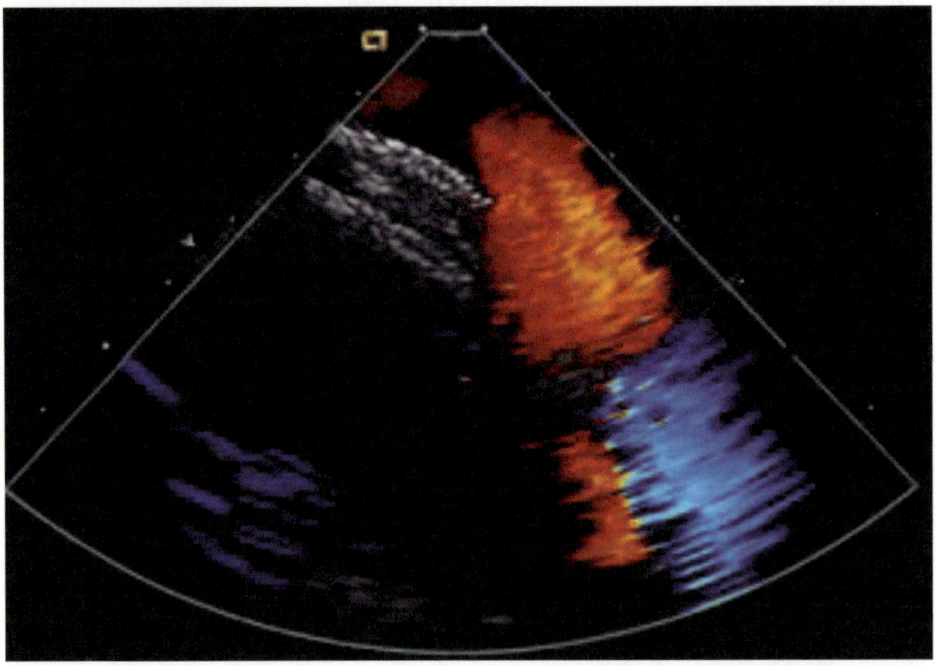

Image 9. Doppler image of a successfully deployed PFO occluder, with significant reduction in the interatrial shunt and no obstruction of the superior vena cava flow.

the PFO was not responsible for the index event, in cases where small emboli formed on the left side of the device, or in cases where closure is incomplete (Wahl, Meier, Haxel et al.,

2001). Thrombosis on the device has been found in about 6% of devices used for PFO closure at one month TEE control in 1000 patients, except for the Amplatzer PFO occluder where it was found in less than 1% (Khairy, O'Donnell & Landzberg 2003).

Pooling the results of the published studies on percutaneous PFO closure, it appears that the intervention yields favorable clinical results over the conservative treatment. Until recently, what came closest to a randomized trial was a matched control follow up study in about 300 patients, of which half were arbitrarily sent for PFO closure by neurologists and half were treated conservatively by the same physicians. Already at a follow up of four years, there was a trend in favor of device closure with an average of 5% events per year (counting all neurological or peripheral symptoms) compared with 7% in the conservative group. This advantage was significant in terms of major strokes, which only occurred in the conservative group. It was also significant in the subgroup of patients who had had more than two events before treatment allocation as well as in those who had complete closure at the six month follow up TEE in the device group (Windecker, Wahl & Nedeltchev, 2004).The few randomized trials in this field have, for years, struggled to enroll sufficient numbers of patients, owing to a variety of factors, including off-label device use.

CLOSURE I

CLOSURE I was the first completed, randomized, and controlled trial comparing the safety and efficacy of percutaneous PFO closure plus medical therapy versus medical therapy alone for secondary TIA and stroke prevention in patients with PFO (CLOSURE I Trial, 2010). CLOSURE I enrolled 909 patients randomized equally to PFO closure using the STARFlex closure device (NMT Medical, Inc. - Boston, MA) as well as six months of aspirin and clopidogrel (and an additional 18 months of aspirin) or to best medical therapy—aspirin or warfarin or a combination. The original endpoint was the 2-year rate of TIA, stroke, or death. Based on a conservative estimate of the expected event rate (6%) from the literature available before 2003, CLOSURE I was originally designed to enroll 1600 patients. However, after 4 years (2003–2006), CLOSURE I had recruited only 611 patients. In April 2007, the FDA approved a proposed revision to the statistical plan that decreased the sample size from 1600 to 800 patients based on an expected event rate of 6% in the medical arm and 2% in the device arm. Patients with cryptogenic TIA or stroke within 6 months and a PFO were screened for study eligibility under the direction of a treating neurologist. To be included, a PFO must have been documented by TEE and amenable to percutaneous closure with STARFlex. For patients randomized to the device arm, the STARFlex device was implanted via percutaneous intervention. The implant procedure was scheduled as soon as possible from the point of randomization, preferably within 1 week. Either TEE or ICE was used during placement of the device.

In the device arm, patients followed a standardized antiplatelet regimen of clopidogrel 75 mg daily for 6 months plus aspirin for the duration of the trial. Patients randomized to medical therapy were treated with one of the following medications throughout the duration of the study: (1) warfarin with a target International Normalized Ratio of 2.0 to 3.0 with an ideal target of 2.5; (2) aspirin 325 mg daily; (3) aspirin 81 mg daily only, allowed for documented gastrointestinal intolerance; or (4) aspirin 81 mg daily with warfarin. Clopidogrel, ticlopidine, and aspirin plus extended-release dipyridamole were not allowed in the medical arm. Heparin was permitted during the initial warfarin treatment period to provide sufficient anticoagulation.At two years, the composite primary endpoints, as well as rates of stroke or TIA alone, were no different between groups. An analysis of outcomes according to baseline characteristics, including shunt size or presence/absence of atrial shunts, also found no differences between groups. Both major vascular complications and atrial fibrillation, mostly periprocedural, were significantly more common in the intervention group, but other safety endpoints were no different between study arms. Procedural and technical success rates (no or trace residual leaking) were suboptimal, with only 86.7% percent of PFOs closed at one year. The majority of the adverse events occurred in the device arm during implantation, raising concerns regarding device delivery techniques by the investigators, as this issue has not arisen in larger trials.

REDUCE

REDUCE is an FDA approved prospective, randomized, multicenter, international trial designed to demonstrate the safety and effectiveness of the Gore Helex Septal Occluder for PFO closure in patients with a history of cryptogenic stroke or imaging-confirmed transient ischemic attack. The FDA approved the Gore Helex Septal Occluder for treatment of atrial septal defect in 2006. The ongoing study includes up to 50 investigational sites in the US and Europe. The Gore REDUCE Study investigators aim to address the CLOSURE I limitations by design- all TIAs must be confirmed by neuroimaging studies such as MRI, which will prevent the inclusion of spurious neurological events that are not vascular in origin. Patients with non-cryptogenic strokes or with a substantial burden of vascular risk factors will be excluded from the trial and a uniform medical therapy regimen will be applied for both test and control subjects (The Gore REDUCE Clinical Study "HLX 06-03").

RESPECT

The RESPECT trial is a randomized, multi-center study investigating whether closure of PFOs using the AMPLATZER PFO Occluder device is safe and effective compared to current standard-of-care treatment in the prevention of a cryptogenic stroke. The RESPECT trial started recruiting patients in 2003 and completed enrollment in January 2012. According to St Jude, RESPECT has enrolled 980 patients over its eight years running, yielding more than 2300 patient-years of data.

The trial is designed to continue until sufficient events have accumulated to be able to assess treatment effectiveness. By protocol, patients enrolled in the trial will continue to be followed until regulatory approval is granted by the FDA, thus providing substantial long-term follow-up on this patient population (RESPECT PFO Clinical Trial).

2. Conclusion

The indication for PFO closure in the face of paradoxical embolism has been widely accepted in the presence of an atrial septal aneurysm or after several embolic events, outside the United States.

Some clinicians choose to close patent foramen ovale in patients with high-risk features, such as stroke despite adequate aspirin or warfarin therapy, large right-to- left interatrial shunts or presence of atrial septal aneurysm.

If the current randomized clinical trials will favor device closure in the setting of paradoxical embolism, it is likely that percutaneous PFO closure will increase significantly in the United States.

3. References

ACC/AHA 2008 Guidelines for the Management of Adults with Congenital Heart Disease. A Report of the American College of Cardiology/American Heart Association Task Force on Practice Guidelines

Bridges ND, Hellenbrand W, Latson L, et al (1992). Transcatheter closure of patent foramen ovale after presumed paradoxical embolism. *Circulation* (86) 1902-1908, 1992.

CLOSURE I Trial (2010)-A Prospective, Multicenter, Randomized, Controlled Trial to Evaluate the Safety and Efficacy of the STARFlex Septal Closure System Versus Best Medical Therapy in Patients With Stroke or Transient Ischemic Attack Due to Presumed Paradoxical Embolism Through a Patent Foramen Ovale. *AHA Scientific Sessions* 2010

Cramer SC, Rordorf G, Maki JH, et al (2004). Increased pelvic vein thrombi in cryptogenic stroke: results of the Paradoxical Emboli from Large Veins in Ischemic Stroke (PELVIS) study. *Stroke* 2004; 35:46 –50.

Deborah R. Gersony, MD, Sang H. Kim, et al (2001): Acute Myocardial Infarction Caused by Paradoxical Coronary Embolization in a Patient with a Patent Foramen Ovale. *J Am Soc Echocardiogr* 2001, 14:1227-9.

DeBelder MA, Towikis L, Leach G, et al. (1992). Risk of patent foramen ovale for thromboembolic events in all age groups. *Am J Cardiol* (69) 1316-1320, 1992.

DiTullio M, Sacco RL, Gopal A, et al. (1992). Patent foramen ovale as a risk factor for cryptogenic stroke. *Ann Intern Med* (117) 461-465, 1992.

GORE HELEX™ Septal Occluder for Patent Foramen Ovale (PFO) Closure in Stroke Patients - The Gore REDUCE Clinical Study "HLX 06-03". NCT00738894 *clinicaltrials.gov*

Hagen PT, Scholz DG, Edwards WD (1984). Incidence and size of patent foramen ovale during the first 10 decades of life: an autopsy study of 965 normal hearts. *Mayo Clin Proc* 1984; 59:17–20.

Hart RG, Miller VT (1983). Cerebral infarctions in young adults: a practical approach. *Stroke* (14) 110-114, 1983.Heart Disease and Stroke Statistics 2009 Update - *American Heart Association*.

Homma S, Sacco RL, Di Tullio MR, Sciacca RR, Mohr JP (2002). Effect of medical treatment in stroke patients with patent foramen ovale: patent foramen ovale in Cryptogenic Stroke Study. *Circulation* 2002; 105:2625–31.

Khairy P, O'Donnell CP, Landzberg MJ (2003). Transcatheter closure versus medical therapy of patent foramen ovale and presumed paradoxical thromboemboli: a systematic review. *Ann Intern Med* 2003; 139:753–60.

King TD, Thompson SL, Steiner C, Mills NL (1976). Secundum atrial septal defect: nonoperative closure during cardiac catheterization. *JAMA* 1976; 235:2506–2509.

Knauth M, Ries S, Pohimann S, et al (1997). Cohort study of multiple brain lesions in sport divers: role of a patent foramen ovale. *BMJ* 1997; 314:701–705.

Kramer, P. (2010). The CardioSEAL/STARFlex family of devices for closure of atrial level defects. In: Transcatheter closure of ASDs and PFOs: A comprehensive assessment, Z. M. Hijazi, T. Feldman, M. H. Abdullah A Al-Qbandi, & H. Sievert *Cardiotext*, Minneapolis, MN, USA, (Eds): 483-399,

Krizanic, F.; Krizanic, F.; Sievert, H.; et al. (2010). The Occlutech Figulla PFO and ASD Occluder: A New Nitinol Wire Mesh Device for Closure of Atrial Septal Defects. *J Invasive Cardiol*, Vol. 22, No. 4, pp. 182–187

Krumsdorf U, Ostermayer S, Billinger K, et al (2004). Incidence and clinical course of thrombus formation on atrial septal defect and patient foramen ovale closure devices in 1,000 consecutive patients. *J Am Coll Cardiol* 2004; 43:302–9.Landefeld CS, Goldman L (1989). Major bleeding in outsubjects treated with warfarin: Incidence and prediction by factors known at the start of outpatient therapy. *Am J Med* 1989 (87) 144-152.

Lamy C, Giannesini C, Zuber M, et al (2002). Clinical and imaging findings in cryptogenic stroke patients with and without patent foramen ovale: the PFO-ASA Study. Atrial septal aneurysm. *Stroke* 2002; 33:706 –11.

Latson, L.; Zahn, E. & Wilson N. (2000). HELEX septal occluder for closure of atrial septal defects. *Curr Intervent Cardiol Rep*, Vol. 2, No. 3, pp. 268-273

Lechat P, Mas JL, Lascault G, et al (1988). Prevalence of patent foramen ovale in patients with stroke. *N Engl J Med* 1988; 318:1148 –52.

Levine M, Hirsch J (2001). Hemorrhagic complications of long term anticoagulant therapy for ischemic vascular disease. *Stroke* 1986 ; (17) 111-116.

Mas JL, Arquizan C, Lamy C, et al (2001). Recurrent cerebrovascular events associated with patent foramen ovale, atrial septal aneurysm, or both. *N Engl J Med* 2001; 345: 1740–6.

Masura, J.; Gavora, P.; Formanek, A. & Hijazi, Z. M. (1997). Transcatheter closure of secundum atrial septal defects using the new self-centering Amplatzer septal occluder: initial human experience. *Cathet Cardiovasc Diagn*, Vol. 42, No. 4, pp. 388-393.

Meier B (2005). Closure of patent foramen ovale: technique, pitfalls, complications, and follow up *Heart* 2005; 91:444–448.

Mohr JP, Thompson JL, Lazar RM, et al (2001). A comparison of warfarin and aspirin for the prevention of recurrent ischemic stroke. *N Engl J Med* 2001; 345:1444 –51.

Moehring MA, Spencer MP (2002). Power M-mode Doppler (PMD) for observing cerebral blood flow and tracking emboli. *Ultrasound Med Biol* 2002; 28:49 –57

Numan M., El Sisi A., et al. (2008). Cribriform Amplatzer Device Closure of Fenestrated Atrial Septal Defects: Feasibility and Technical Aspects. *PediatrCardiol* (2008) 29:530-53.

P Agostoni, G Gasparini, G Destro (2004). Acute myocardial infarction probably caused by paradoxical embolus in a pregnant woman. *Heart* 2004; 90:e12.

Rashkind WJ (1983). Transcatheter treatment of congenital heart disease. *Circulation* 1983; 67: 711–716.

Rosamond W, Flegal K, Friday G, et al. (2007). Heart disease and stroke statistics -- 2007 update: a report from the American Heart Association Statistics Committee and Stroke Statistics Subcommittee. *Circulation* 2007; 115:e69--e171.

RESPECT PFO Clinical Trial-Randomized Evaluation of Recurrent Stroke Comparing PFO Closure to Established Current Standard of Care Treatment. NCT00465270 *clinicaltrials.gov*

Sacco RL, Ellenberg JH, Mohr JP, Tatemichi TK, Hier DB, Price TR, Wolf PA (1989). Infarcts of Undetermined Origin: NINCDS Stroke Data Bank. *Ann Neurol* (25) 382-390, 1989.

Steiner MM, Di Tullio MR, Rundek T, et al. (1998). Patent foramen ovale size and embolic brain imaging findings among patients with ischemic stroke. *Stroke* 1998; 29:944–8.

Schneider B, Hofmann T, Justen MH, Meinertz T (1995). Chiari's network: normal anatomic variant or risk factor for arterial embolic events? *J Am Coll Cardiol* 1995; 26:203–10.

Sloan MA, Alexandrov AV, Tegeler CH, et al. (2004). Assessment: Transcranial Doppler ultrasonography: report of the Therapeutics and Technology Assessment Subcommittee of the American Academy of Neurology. *Neurology* 2004; 62: 1468–81.

Spencer MP, Moehring MA, Jesurum J, Gray WA, Olsen JV, Reisman M (2004). Power M-mode transcranial Doppler for diagnosis of patent foramen ovale and assessing transcatheter closure. *J Neuroimaging* 2004; 14:342–9.

Schwerzmann M, Seiler C, Lipp E, et al (2001). Relation between directly detected patent foramen ovale and ischemic brain lesions in sport divers. *Ann Intern Med* 2001; 134:21–24.

Stroke prevention in Atrial Fibrillation Study: Final Results (1991). *Circulation* 1991 (84) 527-539.

Sideris EB, Sideris SE, Fowlkes JP, et al (1990). Transvenous atrial septal defect occlusion in piglets with a "buttoned" double-disk device. *Circulation* 1990; 81:312–318.

Webster MW, Chancellor AM, Smith HJ, et al. (1988). Patent foramen ovale in young stroke subjects. *Lancet* (8601) 11-12, 1988.

Windecker S, Wahl A, Chatterjee T, et al (2000). Percutaneous closure of patent foramen ovale in patients with paradoxical embolism: long-term risk of recurrent thromboembolic events. *Circulation* 2000;101:893–898.

Wahl A, Meier B, Haxel B, et al (2001). Prognosis after percutaneous closure of patent foramen ovale for paradoxical embolism. *Neurology* 2001; 57:1330–1332.

Windecker S, Wahl A, Nedeltchev K, et al (2004). Comparison of medical treatment with percutaneous closure of patent foramen ovale in patients with cryptogenic stroke. *J Am Coll Cardiol* 2004; 44:750–8.